THE
YOUNG
FOREVER
COOKBOOK

Books by Mark Hyman, MD

Young Forever

The Pegan Diet

Food Fix

Food: What the Heck Should I Cook?

Food: What the Heck Should I Eat?

The Eat Fat, Get Thin Cookbook

Eat Fat, Get Thin

The Blood Sugar Solution 10-Day Detox Diet Cookbook

The Blood Sugar Solution 10-Day Detox Diet

The Blood Sugar Solution Cookbook

The Blood Sugar Solution

The Daniel Plan

The Daniel Plan Cookbook

UltraPrevention

UltraMetabolism

The Five Forces of Wellness (CD)

The UltraMetabolism Cookbook

The UltraThyroid Solution

The UltraSimple Diet

The UltraMind Solution

Six Weeks to an UltraMind (CD)

UltraCalm (CD)

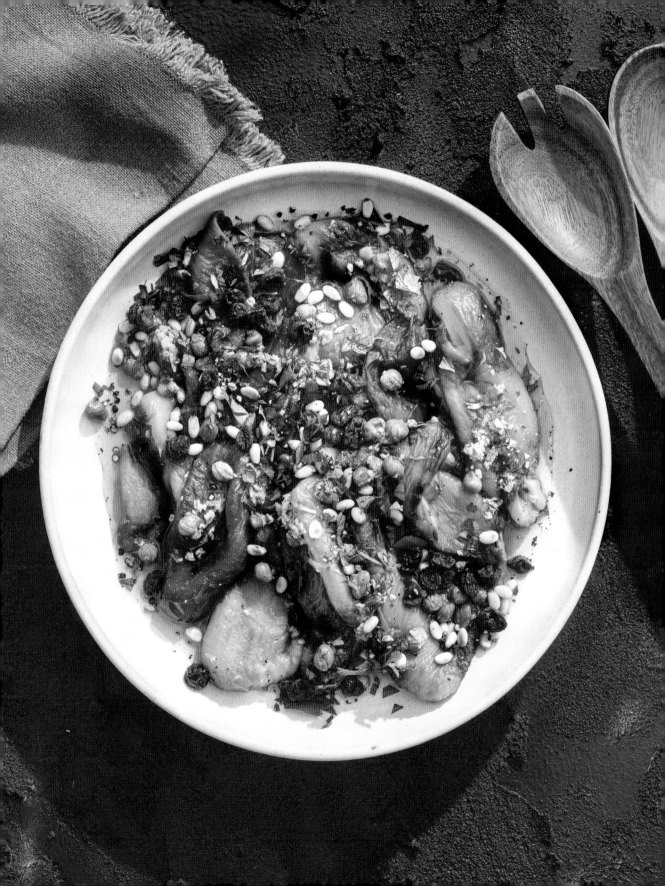

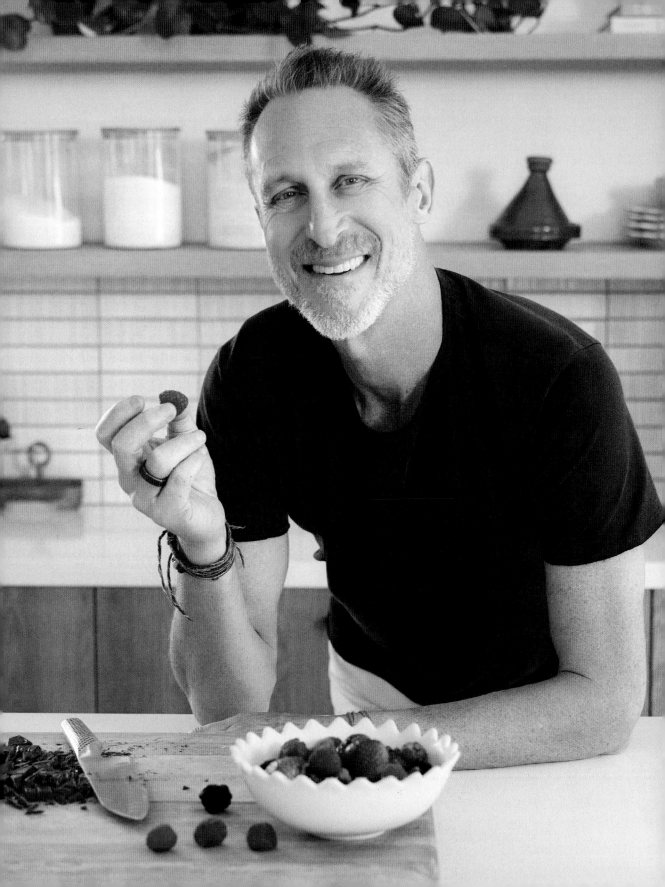

THE
YOUNG
FOREVER

COOKBOOK

**MORE THAN 100 DELICIOUS RECIPES FOR
LIVING YOUR LONGEST, HEALTHIEST LIFE**

Mark Hyman, MD

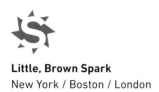

Little, Brown Spark
New York / Boston / London

Little, Brown Spark
Hachette Book Group
1290 Avenue of the Americas, New York, NY 10104
littlebrownspark.com

First Edition: June 2024

Little, Brown Spark is an imprint of Little, Brown and Company, a division of Hachette Book Group, Inc. The Little, Brown Spark name and logo are trademarks of Hachette Book Group, Inc.

The publisher is not responsible for websites (or their content) that are not owned by the publisher.

The Hachette Speakers Bureau provides a wide range of authors for speaking events. To find out more, go to hachettespeakersbureau.com or email HachetteSpeakers@hbgusa.com.

Little, Brown and Company books may be purchased in bulk for business, educational, or promotional use. For information, please contact your local bookseller or the Hachette Book Group Special Markets Department at special.markets@hbgusa.com.

Recipes
Food stylist and culinary consultant: Dara Sutin
Photographer: Kyla Zanardi
Prop stylist and art director: Rayna Marlee Schwartz
Recipe tester and food styling assistant: Becca Pozner

Photographs of Dr. Mark Hyman
Photographer: Masha Maltsava
Food stylist: Jessica Boone

Interior design by Empire Design Studio

ISBN 978-0-316-57162-3

LCCN 2023949234

10 9 8 7 6 5 4 3 2 1

LSC-C

Printed in Canada

*To the dreamers and seekers and adventurers who imagine
a life without chronic disease, who are searching for
a way to live a long and healthy life*

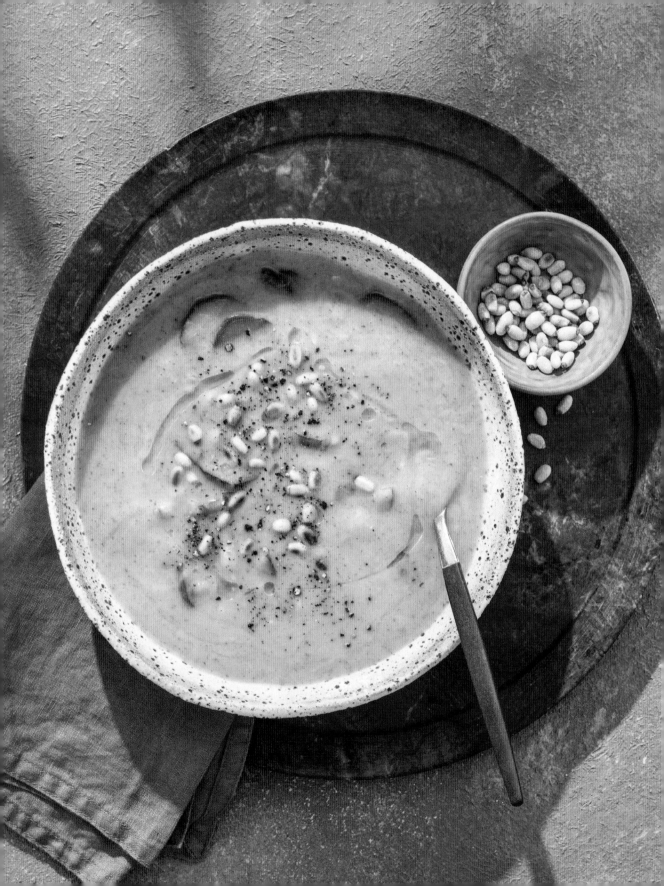

CONTENTS

The fountain of youth is within reach for all of us. It's quite simple. You might want to seek out the latest scientific discoveries to help extend your health span and lifespan, but the true answer is found in places known as the Blue Zones, where life has remained mostly unchanged for a thousand years, where there are twenty times as many centenarians as we have in America. People in the Blue Zones practice ancient foodways and have a deep sense of community, belonging, purpose, and meaning. I traveled to a few of those places and saw, smelled, and tasted the joy of simple food shared in community.

One of the Blue Zones is a Sardinian mountain area that has changed little over the past millennium, a place where ancient methods of growing, preserving, preparing, and sharing food have been preserved. The inhabitants all have gardens ripe with tomatoes, peppers, eggplants, chard, artichokes, blackberries, and strawberries, and orchards of figs, chestnuts, pomegranates, and almonds. They live with their animals—goats, sheep, pigs, and chickens—and they understand that what they feed the animals affects their flavor. They know that certain wild and cultivated plants make their milk, cheese, and meat taste better. These plants also happen to be rich in healing phytochemicals.

When I first arrived in Sardinia, we went to Olinto Fantozzi's farm for lunch, which was more like a feast. Olinto, a jovial and enthusiastic sixty-year-old, served us a nose-to-tail meal from his pigs—the head, cheeks, lungs, heart, liver, intestines, and meat. He told us about the wild plants, acorns, and ancient grains the animals are fed—the flavor comes from seasoning the meat *before* the animal is killed. We drank his Cannonau wine and gentian grappa and ate his rabbits and almond-honey nougat, his plethora of summer tomatoes of all sizes and colors, and his olives seasoned with local herbs of thyme and bay leaves. We ate his homemade culurgiones, little pierogi-like dumplings made from an ancient form of wheat, grano cappelli, and stuffed with potato and sheep cheese. We ate his goat cheeses and preserved meats from different parts of the pig. He proudly shared his aged goat cheese made with worms—a natural Viagra, he said. According to family legend, his grandmother fed his grandfather this cheese before he died, and she was able to have sex with him right up until he passed away! I braved a bite, worms included!

Olinto took us on a tour of his olive, fig, apricot, peach, and apple orchards; his simple garden of eggplants, peppers, zucchini, and tomatoes; and his chickens, pigs, sheep, and rabbits. All of this on land his family has owned for centuries, in a house of stone he built himself, on a rugged mountainside where he lived alone, happily tending to his animals, his land, and the few who come to share meals at his old wooden table. Joyously, he celebrates his life, his land, his food, and his cooking. Government food regulations have made it almost impossible for him to prepare food in the ancient ways—with rules about raw milk and butchering—and though he may skirt some of these rules, his food *gives* life while the "approved" food, he says, makes everyone sick and fat.

While we all can't pack up and move to remote lands, growing our own food and herding our sheep and goats, we can apply a few longevity lessons from the Blue Zones:

- Eat food grown in ways that increase its nutrient density—organically and naturally.

- Eat animals that are raised in ways that are humane.

- Restore the soil, water, and ecosystem to create a nutrient-rich source of protein. (The healthier the soil and thusly plants grown from it, the healthier the animals that feed on these plants.)

- Eat mostly plants. Keep meat as a side dish. Quality should be your North Star when shopping, cooking, and eating.

- Learn to find joy in cooking and preparing life-giving meals to share with loved ones.

- Find connectedness and camaraderie in community. Sharing in life with others is as old as we are as a species.

We have lost our connection to the source of our food. We have lost ancient traditions. Cooking from scratch is a vanishing art. The food industry has imposed itself on our kitchens, providing an endless array of tantalizing colors, sizes, and shapes of addictive, processed food–like substances that drive our epidemic of chronic disease, obesity, and rapid aging. The keys to health and longevity are found on the farm, at the grocery store, and in your kitchen.

As a child, I grew up knowing where my food came from. My mother and father left America for Europe in the early 1950s before food became industrialized, before the American kitchen revolved around convenience food, food that inconveniently makes us sick and shortens our life. My mother shopped in the local markets in Barcelona, where I was born. There was no supermarket, just small specialty shops. The fruit and vegetables stand, the butcher, the baker. There was no real refrigeration, only a small ice box, so fresh food was purchased (and available) daily. Back home in the suburbs in the 1970s, while much of America was being sold on Tang, Pop-Tarts, Fleischmann's margarine, and Swanson TV dinners, my mother grew a garden in our backyard with tomatoes, zucchini, cucumbers, lettuces, and herbs, and cultivated a small orchard of plum, pear, and apple trees. She followed the advice of my grandmother Mary: "Buy fresh, eat fresh." We ate family dinners together every night, meals of simple, real food made from scratch.

As a young adult, I lived with a group of other college students who cared about food and where it came from. We ripped up the lawn in the backyard and planted a garden. We sourced maple syrup by tapping the trees along the street where we lived. We shopped at the farmers' market and belonged to the local food co-op, where we bought our grains, beans, nuts, seeds, oils, spices, and other food from bulk bins. We cooked delicious meals every night and shared them in community. It was during this time that I honed my skills in the kitchen and learned to cook for large groups. My mother always said to me, "If you can read, you can cook," and I followed recipes that taught me the basic principles of cooking. Seeking out delicious whole ingredients and preparing meals for my family and friends has turned into my greatest joy.

And now, as a physician, my mission is to apply the lessons I have learned throughout my life to help my patients heal and create lives absent of disease. If food is medicine, then this cookbook is the prescription pad. The recipes in this book are your doctor's order for health and longevity. Enjoy them, experiment with them, create health from them. It is my hope that you use this cookbook to learn your way around the kitchen, to invite friends over and enlist them in cooking, to share the ritual of mealtime with your community, to create a rich, meaningful connection to food and health that begins in the kitchen. This is the medicine we need to heal much of what is ailing us—individually and as a society.

SETTING UP
FOR SUCCESS

The single most important thing you do each day is eat. What you eat matters. Food is not just nourishment or pleasure. It provides instructions that can upgrade or downgrade your biology with every bite. Food is medicine, literally. It is the stuff we are made of, the stuff that regulates every aspect of our biology from our immune system to our hormones, brain chemistry, gene expression, and even our microbiome. It is the key to living a long healthy life.

Making the right choices can be difficult. We live in a food carnival, a toxic nutritional landscape where making the right choices is hard and making the wrong choices is easy. We are busy, stretched, and pulled in many directions: family, work, endless to-do lists. But it's important to eat well, in a way that can extend both your health span and your lifespan. Ground zero for your health just happens to be as close as your kitchen.

Food, real whole food, contains thousands of molecules. Yes, protein, fat, and carbs; fiber, vitamins, and minerals. But also, tens of thousands of phytonutrients that interact with your biology, controlling critical processes that keep you healthy. Many of the ancient built-in survival systems encoded in your genes depend on the right balance of nutrients to thrive. Food has the power to activate these systems of renewal, repair, and regeneration. Choosing what you eat is the most consequential act for your health and well-being. And this might look different for everyone.

There is no one perfect way of eating for everyone. Your genetics, culture, taste preferences, beliefs, and health challenges shape your dietary choices. However, whether you're an omnivore, paleo, vegetarian, or vegan, here are simple guidelines you can follow to optimize your nutrient intake, increase your energy, feel healthier, and maybe even live longer:

- Eat real food.
- Focus on quality and nutrient density.
- Avoid ultra-processed food.
- Keep sugar and starch to a minimum.
- Eat lots of plants.
- Ensure you consume enough omega-3 fats.
- Eat enough high-quality protein to maintain your muscle mass.

Your health starts in your kitchen, not in your doctor's office. When you reclaim your kitchen by purging industrial food-like substances, filling it with real food, and learning simple cooking techniques, you will be on the path to a long and healthy life.

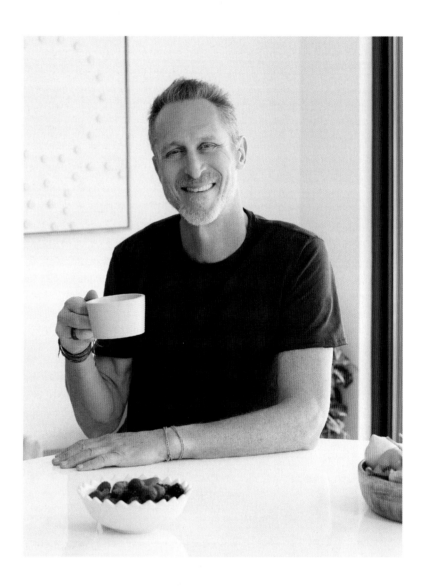

FUELING UP

The key to establishing a healthy routine at home begins in your kitchen. Avoiding highly processed, packaged foods and leaning into homemade alternatives that are more satiating and nutritious are the first steps in building the foundation for better health. For millennia, nutritional wisdom was passed from generation to generation. But over the last sixty years, the food industry has hijacked the American kitchen and out-sourced cooking to factories. This has led to an explosion of weight gain, obesity, and chronic disease and has shortened our life expectancy for the first time in history. It is time to reclaim our kitchens and our health.

Be smart in the grocery store and kitchen. Think of your grocery store as your "farmacy" and choose foods that are the best medicine for your body. Read packaging labels. If a label lists ingredients you recognize—for instance, a can of tomatoes lists water, tomatoes, and salt—the food is fine. If it lists industrial ingredients, or words you can't pronounce or don't recognize as food (such as maltodextrin or partially hydrogenated fats), or additives, preservatives, or artificial flavors, put that food back on the shelf. It has no place in your kitchen or your body.

Choose real ingredients. Vegetables, fruit, nuts, seeds, traditional oils such as olive oil, whole grains and beans, and spices. Opt for clean proteins, if possible those that are regeneratively raised, grass-fed, pasture-raised, or organic. Buy rainbow-colored vegetables and fruit; they contain phytonutrients that regulate ancient biological pathways designed to keep you healthy, reduce inflammation, fertilize your microbiome, and control your "longevity switches."

LEARN TO BECOME A BETTER COOK

Most people know they need to eat healthier, but they don't know where to start. The recipes in this book are designed to include health-promoting foods and ingredients that will maximize your potential to live a long and healthy life. Did you know, for instance, that eating more nuts and seeds can lower your risk of heart disease and diabetes? Or that the zinc in pumpkin seeds can boost your immune system and digestion?

Straightforward, healthful, and delicious, these recipes will help you gain confidence in your cooking skills and allow you to be creative with meal planning. Choosing food in the grocery store, handling it, cleaning it, prepping it, and cooking it are acts that make us human. Practicing cooking is easy and fun, and cooking with your family or friends, savoring food together, is something we humans have been doing since the dawn of time.

You don't need to be a master chef to prepare tasty, nutrient-dense foods at home. The simple techniques and recipes in this book will inspire you to experiment with new flavors and become more comfortable with cooking. You may want to prepare a quick, easy meal after a long day's work, or a more festive meal that takes a little more time. Either way, there's a recipe here for you.

Here are some tips to help you become a more self-assured home cook:

- **Practice the mise en place.** Taken from the French term meaning *put in place*, this is the key to creating a successful dish. It means having your ingredients prepped, tools and equipment at the ready, and everything organized before you even start cooking.

- **Understand your ingredients.** Never seen a kohlrabi before? New to spatchcocking a whole chicken? Working with new ingredients or techniques can be daunting. Don't fret. I will guide you, mapping out the best way to tackle a new vegetable or learn the easiest way to prepare a cut of meat. Learning as we go is the best chef's education.

- **Give yourself extra time.** Following a recipe can be as simple as taking one step at a time. However, if you are new to cooking, each step might take a bit longer than expected. Rather than feeling rushed or confined by the suggested cooking time, allow yourself extra time for prepping the food, putting it together, and cooking it so you can approach each new recipe with confidence.

- **Learn to trust yourself.** These recipes are just that, recipes. They are not set in stone, merely guidelines on how to prepare certain foods. Using your gut or intuition is key to becoming a great cook. Taste your food as it's cooking to understand the balance between sweet, savory, and acidic. Perhaps your oven runs hot; you can already smell the caramelization on the vegetables, so it's time to take them out. Learning to cook like this, using all your senses, is the most natural way to instill confidence. It takes time, but it is a journey worth embarking on.

- **Have fun!** Think of preparing home-cooked meals as a pleasure rather than a chore. Think of cooking as an art. Every time you step into the kitchen, you have a chance to be creative, to feel, touch, and smell the very sustenance for life. Learn, experiment, play, put on music, gather your family and friends. Make something yummy and healing.

Learning to prepare fresh meals with real whole ingredients will delight your senses and your biology. It is time to activate your body's ancient healing and survival pathways, your longevity switches. The recipes in this book range from easy, wholesome snacks to nutrient-dense dinners. I hope they inspire you to reclaim your kitchen and get cooking. The side effect? Renewed energy, well-being, disease reversal, and longevity.

STOCKING YOUR PANTRY

The key to becoming a successful home cook and preparing recipes that are nutrient-dense, flavorful, and healthy, is to stock your pantry well. Having a well-curated selection of ingredients on hand is the first step to creating truly delicious meals. Cooking becomes easy when you're prepared.

I cook with whole, real food. Fresh produce, wild-caught fish and seafood, grass-fed beef and lamb, pasture-raised poultry, pasture-raised eggs, and organic pantry staples. Increasingly these foods are available in grocery stores and online, making it easier to eat well. It is important to learn which foods heal and which harm. Health claims on labels such as gluten- or dairy-free products often disguise other harmful ingredients. However, there is a whole array of healthy options for gluten-, dairy-, and sugar-free foods for those who need them. Larger grocers such as Walmart, Costco, and Trader Joe's, and online sources of whole food such as Thrive Market, Seatopia.fish (for regeneratively raised fish), and Force of Nature (for regeneratively raised meat) make it much more affordable to eat food that is delicious, good for you, and good for the planet.

The key is to stock your kitchen with the right building blocks for creating tasty, life-giving meals. Here are some key items you'll want to have on hand.

OILS

Not all oils are created equal. Many common cooking oils, such as refined seed and bean oils, are inflammatory and can cause negative impacts on our health. I've done the research for you. Following is a list of oils I use at home. They are healthful, delicious, and easily accessible. They should be cold-pressed and organic.

Avocado oil	*MCT oil*
Coconut oil	*Olive oil, extra virgin (for dressings, finishing)*
Hazelnut oil or walnut oil	*Sesame oil, toasted*

VINEGARS

Vinegar is an important acid for your kitchen. Unlike lemon or lime juice, vinegar results from fermentation by acetic acid, which can heighten other flavors and balance out the sweetness or saltiness in a dish. It can be made from a variety of ingredients, producing unique characteristics that add vibrancy and flavor. Following are some of my favorite vinegars. Be sure to check the labels for no added sugars.

Apple cider vinegar

Balsamic vinegar

Red wine vinegar

Rice wine vinegar

Sherry vinegar

White wine vinegar

CONDIMENTS AND SAUCES

Condiments and sauces can add flavor to any dish. Often excellent sources of umami—the fifth taste that we can sense—condiments and sauces only need to be used sparingly to really have an impact.

Coconut aminos (without colorings and sweeteners)

Fish sauce

Gochujang paste

Harissa paste

Kimchi

Miso, white (organic and gluten-free)

Mustard, Dijon and grainy Dijon

Soy sauce (low-sodium)

Sriracha

Tahini

Tamari (gluten-free)

CANNED GOODS

These cooking essentials are always in my pantry. They are nonperishable and inexpensive, adding flavor, texture, and nutrients to any dish.

Anchovies

Beans (cannellini, chickpeas, black-eyed peas, black beans, navy beans, lentils, etc.)

Capers

Chipotles in adobo

Coconut milk (full-fat unsweetened)

Olives, kalamata and Castelvetrano

Salmon, wild (sustainably caught)

Sardines (wild-caught)

Stock, chicken (organic and/or pasture-raised)

Stock, vegetable (organic)

Tomatoes, diced

Tomatoes, whole peeled

Tomato paste

ALTERNATIVE FLOURS, GRAINS, NUTS, AND SEEDS

Many of these ingredients may be new to you, but it's worth experimenting with them. They are highly nutritious and delicious. Some of the gluten-free ingredients listed below are great alternatives to the traditional highly processed flours and foods we often see in recipes.

One tip: I like to keep my raw nuts and seeds in the freezer to prevent them from spoiling.

Almonds, ground

Arrowroot powder

Buckwheat, Himalayan Tartary (from Big Bold Health)

Buckwheat groats

Cacao powder, raw (unsweetened)

Coconut, shredded, flakes, and desiccated (unsweetened)

Flour, almond

Flour, chickpea

Flour, coconut

Honey (raw, unfiltered)

Lentils, dried

Maple syrup, pure (organic)

Monk fruit sweetener, powdered

Nuts (whole raw almonds, cashews, Brazil nuts)

Nut butters (almond, cashew)

Protein powder, whey or vegan

Quinoa

Rice (black, brown, wild)

Seeds (chia seeds, hemp seeds, pumpkin seeds, white sesame seeds, black sesame seeds, sunflower seeds)

Soba noodles, buckwheat

Sugar, coconut

SPICES AND OTHER FLAVOR ENHANCERS

Spices have antioxidant, antimicrobial, and anti-inflammatory properties and are one of the easiest ways to enhance a dish. Be sure to check your spices after a year or two as they tend to lose their potency.

Aleppo pepper

Cayenne pepper

Chili flakes, red

Chili powder

Cinnamon sticks

Coriander, ground

Coriander seeds

Cumin, ground

Cumin seeds

Salt, kosher (I prefer Diamond brand)

Salt, sea salt flakes

Nori sheets

Paprika, smoked	*Shiitakes, dried*
Paprika, sweet	*Sumac*
Peppercorns, black (or ground black pepper)	*Turmeric*
	Vanilla extract, pure

STAPLES

These are just some of the foods I can't live without! They appear in many of the recipes in this book, so keep them on hand in your kitchen. My philosophy is simple: Eat a rainbow of colors for maximum health. Eat an abundance of fresh greens for their phytochemicals: reds for their carotenoids, which can help prevent cancer; orange for antioxidants like alpha-carotene; and purples for their anthocyanins, which can help prevent aging. Have the right fats available. Choose sheep or goat cheese over cow dairy, and always keep pasture-raised eggs on hand for quick meals. I often keep vacuum-sealed ground bison, chicken, and fish on hand for times I'm in a pinch. Make sure you choose pasture-raised, grass-fed, and organic meats and poultry whenever possible, as well as wild-caught, sustainable, and organic fish and shellfish.

Dairy

Butter (grass-fed)	*Eggs (pasture-raised)*
Cheese, sheep's or goat milk (such as feta or pecorino)	*Yogurt, sheep's milk*

Fruits and Vegetables

Avocados	*Herbs, fresh (parsley, cilantro, mint, thyme)*
Berries, fresh or frozen (blueberries, raspberries)	*Lemons and limes*
Carrots	*Mushrooms (shiitake, cremini)*
Celery	*Onions (yellow, red)*
Chiles (Thai red, jalapeño)	*Scallions*
Garlic	*Shallots*
Ginger	*Squash, winter (butternut, acorn)*
Greens, dark leafy (kale, Swiss chard, baby spinach)	*Sweet potatoes or Japanese purple potatoes*

Meat

Beef, grass-fed

Bison, ground (grass-fed)

Chicken or turkey, ground (pasture-raised)

Fish

Salmon, wild-caught

Shrimp, wild-caught (frozen)

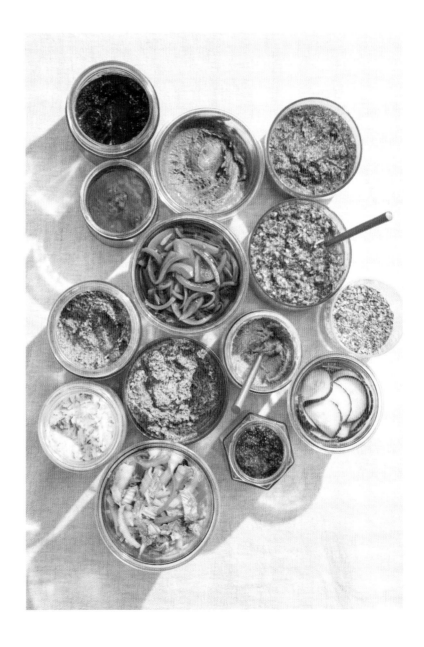

COOKING EQUIPMENT

If you want to cook, you need to have the right tools. Investing in high-quality kitchen tools is an investment in your health. And one you will only need to make once if you choose the right pots and pans, knives, and kitchen accessories. I still have my grandmother's garlic press and a cast-iron pan I got in college forty years ago. Investing a little more up front will ensure you will have them for a lifetime. It also makes cooking easier and more fun.

KNIVES

High-quality, sharp knives are essential. They make cutting and chopping easier, faster, and safer. German brands like Wüsthof make great affordable chef's knives that you can buy almost anywhere. If you're an avid cook wanting to upgrade your set, look for Japanese brands like Shun or Mac. They sell great knives at various price points made from heavy-duty steel with comfortable handles, making chopping tasks easier. You can buy a whole set or start with just three knives that can cover most of the bases. Another favorite is the Victorinox small, serrated knife, great for slicing things like cherry tomatoes and small fruit. The key is to build a collection over time, so start with a small chef's knife (4 to 5 inches) for cutting vegetables and a large chef's knife (about 8 inches) for larger vegetables like squash and onions, and a small, serrated knife.

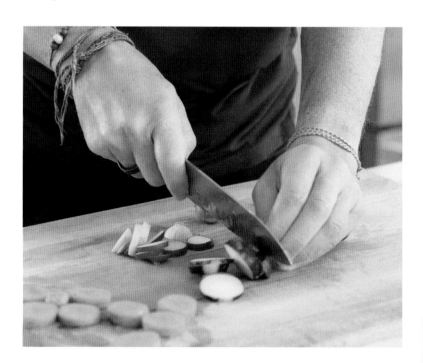

VITAMIX BLENDER

While a Vitamix is not cheap, it will last you a lifetime. It is my most essential kitchen appliance. I use it daily to make smoothies, soups, dips, and sauces. You can find decent blenders at various prices, but they won't last as long as the Vitamix.

FOOD PROCESSOR

There is a big difference between a blender and a food processor. A blender liquifies where a food processor is meant to chop and crush, and often comes with attachments to grate and slice. Use a food processor to grate vegetables, chop salsas, make dips and nut butters, and much more. If you are going to invest in one thing for your kitchen, make it the Cuisinart Custom 14-cup food processor, a heavy-duty machine that will last you a lifetime.

IMMERSION BLENDER

A useful tool if you're not ready to splurge on a blender is a hand-held immersion blender. It is easy to clean, compact, and effective at pureeing, although it won't get your soups as smooth as a blender will. Nevertheless, it's extremely handy for whipping up salad dressings and quick pestos, and it is inexpensive. Cuisinart and Breville make the highest quality hand-held blenders.

GRATERS

I use graters almost every day, and they come in a variety of blade shapes and sizes. I have two or three ranging from fine to coarse and use them for zesting, grating garlic and ginger, and grating cheese. Box graters are a good alternative for grating large vegetables if you don't have a grating attachment on your food processor.

PANS

Invest in high-quality pans that will last a lifetime. Nonstick or stainless steel pans are both great options to have on hand. I like to have a couple sizes of nontoxic, nonstick pans for cooking eggs and searing chicken. My favorite brands for nonstick pans are Scanpan, GreenPan, and All-Clad. I also have a few stainless steel pans, which, when preheated correctly, are completely nonstick and have no coating. You can decide which you prefer to cook with. I highly advise purchasing a large, heavy cast-iron pan; it's great for cooking steak, searing vegetables, and even baking! I also recommend a griddle pan if you don't have access to an outdoor grill.

POTS

You'll need a range of pots in different sizes. Whether you're boiling water, reheating soup, cooking stock, or slowly stewing, you'll be using saucepans and pots every day. It's a good idea to invest in a set of five or six pots, including a saucepan and a stockpot. Again, invest in high-quality stainless steel cookware for best results.

DUTCH OVEN

A classic Dutch oven, or heavy bottomed cast-iron pot fitted with a lid, is a great investment. This pot can do just about anything when it comes to cooking: braising, stewing, searing, and sautéing. The great thing is that Dutch ovens are ovenproof, making them perfect for slow cooking. There are many good-quality cast-iron Dutch ovens on the market at different price ranges. Staub and Le Creuset are at the higher end, while Lodge and Cuisinart are more affordable.

KITCHEN ACCESSORIES

Here is a list of tools I simply can't cook without:

Baking sheets, standard 13x18-inch	*Measuring spoons*
Can opener	*Mixing bowls*
Citrus reamer	*Scissors*
Colander	*Sieve*
Cutting boards (one for animal products, one for fruits and vegetables)	*Silicone spatulas*
	Thermometer, instant-read
Kitchen scale	*Tongs, silicone or metal, two sizes*
Measuring cups (metal or glass)	*Vegetable peeler*
	Wire whisk

These items will make it easier and more fun to cook at home. Having a fully stocked kitchen will set you up for success on the path towards a longer, healthier life!

    Let's get cooking!

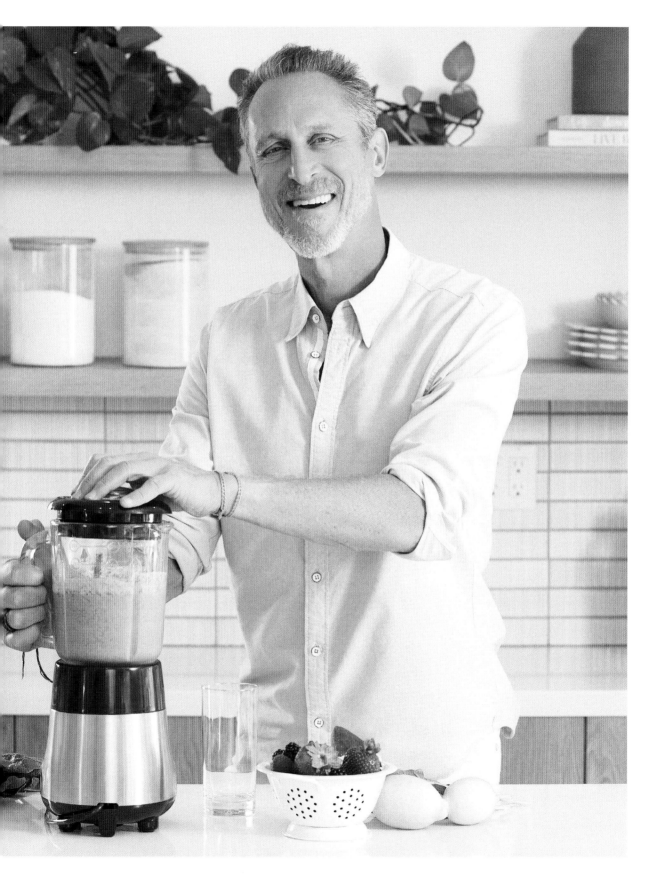

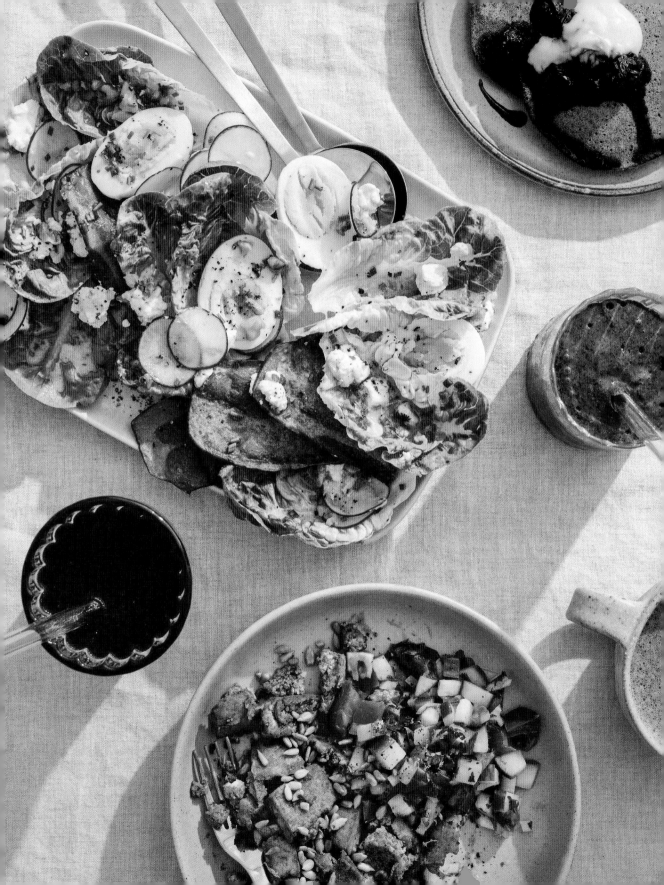

Breakfast

Breakfast is one of the most important meals of the day; we've all heard that saying before. I'm here to tell you, it truly is. Eating a protein-rich, substantial breakfast can help propel your day in the right direction as well as provide adequate nutrition for longevity, fueling your body with essential nutrients like calcium, fiber, and vitamin C. Breakfast doesn't have to be complicated, but it should be the one meal that gets you out of bed in the morning. Whether it's my Ultimate Recovery Smoothie (page 20), lush Baked Eggs with Chickpeas and Tomatoes (page 13), or the best Smoky Scrambled Tofu with Chopped Salad (page 15), these ideas for breakfast are sure to provide flavor, nutrition, and enough variety that you'll have a hard time trying to figure out which to eat first!

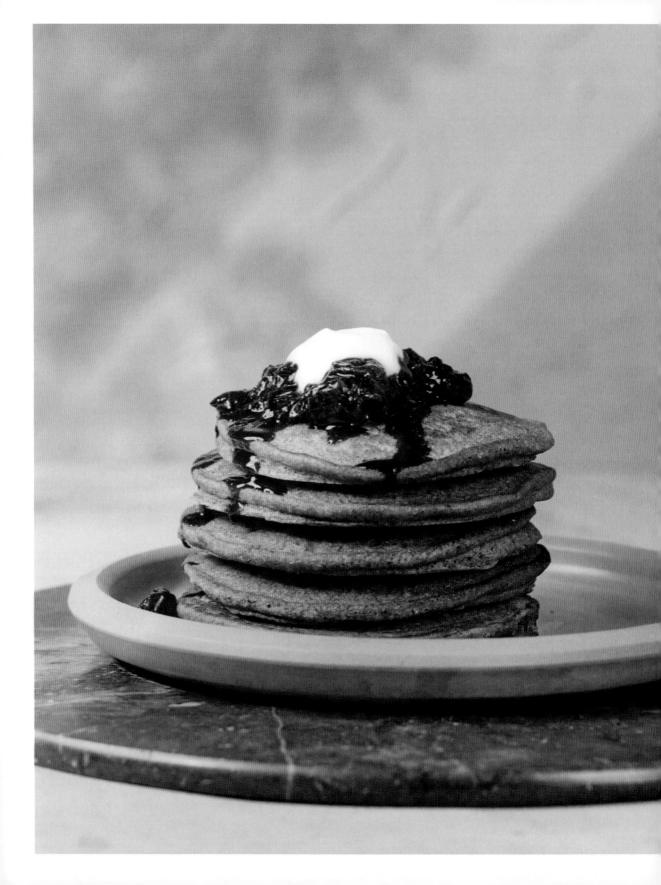

Himalayan Tartary Buckwheat and Berry Pancakes

Serves: 2 to 4

Makes: 10 to 12 pancakes
Prep Time: 10 minutes
Cook Time: 15 minutes

Pancake Batter

1½ cups almond milk (or milk of choice), plus more if needed

2 teaspoons lemon juice or apple cider vinegar

¾ cup Himalayan Tartary buckwheat flour

1 cup almond flour

1 teaspoon baking powder

1 teaspoon ground cinnamon

½ teaspoon ground nutmeg

¼ teaspoon kosher salt

2 large pasture-raised organic eggs, lightly whisked

2 tablespoons maple syrup

1 teaspoon vanilla extract

Compote

2 cups fresh or frozen blueberries

½ cup water

¼ cup orange juice

1 to 2 tablespoons maple syrup or honey (optional)

Grass-fed unsalted butter, for cooking

¼ cup coconut or dairy-free yogurt, for serving

These are not your average pancakes. Made with unique Himalayan Tartary buckwheat flour, they are loaded with phytonutrients, prebiotic fiber, and magnesium, all of which contain significant nutrients for a healthy gut microbiome. As one of the highest antioxidant foods out there, Tartary buckwheat flour contains a unique phytonutrient-dense, immune-supporting compound called Hobamine, which has been linked to slowing down the aging process. Naturally gluten-free, these pancakes are a delicious and nutritious start to your morning.

1. Preheat the oven to 325°F. Line a rimmed baking sheet with a wire rack.

2. **For the pancake batter:** In a large measuring cup, combine 1 cup of the almond milk and lemon juice. Set aside for 5 minutes.

3. In a mixing bowl, whisk together the buckwheat flour, almond flour, baking powder, cinnamon, nutmeg, and salt.

4. Create a well in the center of the dry ingredients and pour in the eggs, almond milk mixture, maple syrup, and vanilla. Whisk together until all the ingredients are incorporated, adding up to ½ cup additional almond milk if the batter is too thick. Be careful not to overbeat; a few lumps are fine.

5. **To make the compote:** Place all the ingredients in a saucepan over medium heat. Bring to a boil, then reduce the heat and simmer for 5 to 10 minutes, until the mixture has thickened. Gently mash the berries with a fork and set aside until you're ready to serve.

6. Heat a nonstick pan or griddle over medium heat. Add some butter to the pan. Working in batches and using a measuring cup, ladle ¼ cup of the batter into the pan, forming one or two pancakes and leaving an inch between them. Cook for 1 to 2 minutes, until small bubbles begin to form on the surface, then flip and continue cooking for another 2 minutes, until golden brown. Transfer the pancakes to the wire rack in the baking sheet and keep warm in the oven as you cook the remaining pancakes.

7. To serve, stack a few pancakes on a plate and top with a heaping spoonful of the berry compote and a dollop of yogurt.

Kimchi, Egg, and Avocado Bowl

Serves: 2

Prep Time: 10 minutes

Cook Time: 10 minutes

1 teaspoon sesame oil

1 garlic clove, thinly sliced

1 large handful green curly kale, deveined and shredded

Pinch of kosher salt

1 tablespoon avocado oil

2 large pasture-raised organic eggs

1 cup cooked grains, such as brown basmati rice or quinoa

½ cup Quick "Kimchi" (page 213) or store-bought kimchi

4 scallions, white and light green parts, thinly sliced

1 avocado, pitted, peeled, and sliced

1 tablespoon toasted sesame seeds

1 tablespoon coconut aminos or gluten-free tamari (optional)

One of my favorite ways to enjoy eggs is with kimchi. An unlikely breakfast component, fermented kimchi is the perfect vinegary complement to creamy avocado and rich egg yolk. This breakfast bowl is infinitely adaptable, and perfect for using up leftovers in the fridge.

1. Heat the sesame oil in a skillet over medium heat. Add the garlic and cook for 1 minute, until lightly golden. Add the kale with a splash of water and cook, stirring, for 4 minutes, until soft. Season with a pinch of salt and remove from the pan; set aside.

2. In the same pan, heat the avocado oil over medium heat. Crack in the eggs and cook for 4 to 5 minutes, until the whites are set and the yolks are warm.

3. Scoop ½ cup of the grains into each of two bowls. Top with kale, kimchi, scallions, avocado, and one egg. Sprinkle with sesame seeds and serve with coconut aminos or tamari if desired.

The Young Forever Cookbook

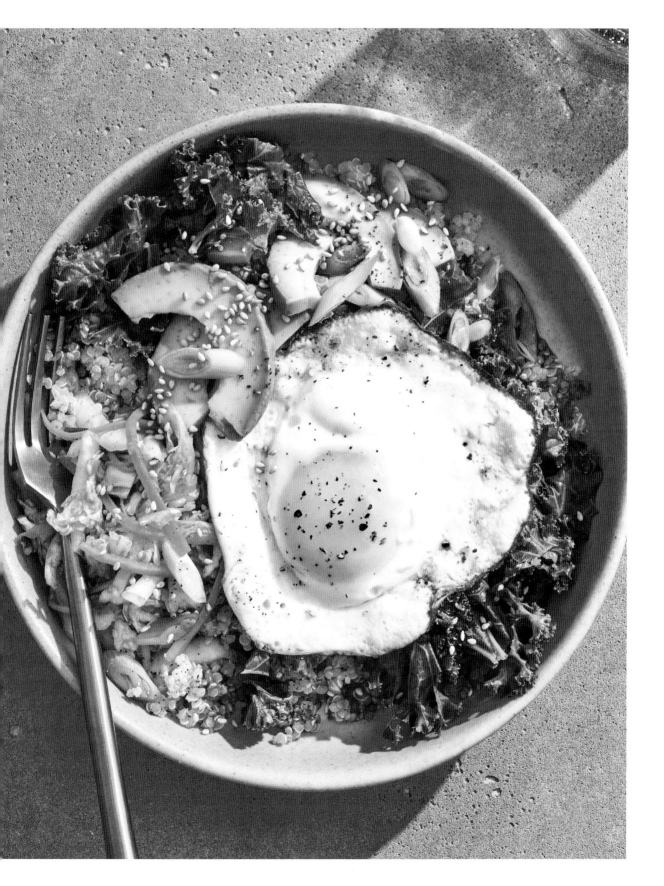

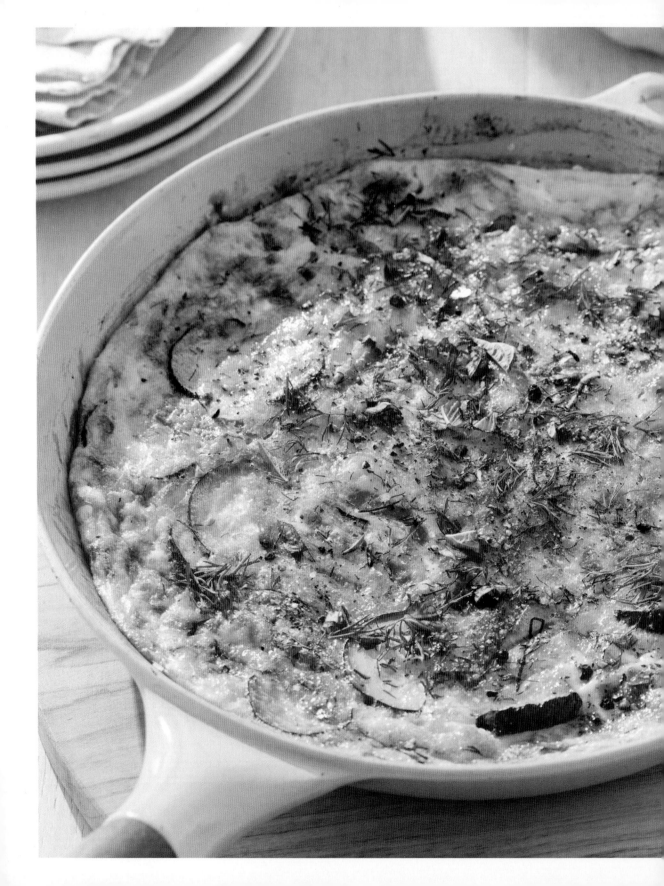

Roasted Red Pepper and Zucchini Frittata

Serves: 4

Prep Time: 15 minutes

Cook Time: 30 minutes

2 tablespoons extra-virgin olive oil

1 yellow onion, thinly sliced

2 garlic cloves, minced

1 large zucchini, halved lengthwise then sliced into half-moons

1½ teaspoons kosher salt

1 cup roasted red peppers from a jar, drained and roughly chopped

2 cups packed baby spinach

8 large pasture-raised organic eggs

⅓ cup finely chopped mixed soft fresh herbs such as basil and dill

¼ cup grated pecorino cheese

½ teaspoon freshly ground black pepper

Frittatas are one of the simplest ways to incorporate vegetables into eggs and a great way to use up what's in your fridge. Yet they are simple to prepare and easily serve a crowd. Sautéed zucchini, red peppers, and baby spinach fill this sturdy and substantial frittata, which is delicious both warm and cold. The recipe can easily handle vegetable swaps of whatever is in season, such as leftover cooked squash and fresh sage for an autumnal version, or fresh cherry tomatoes and basil in the summer.

1. Preheat the broiler to high.

2. Heat the olive oil in a 10-inch ovenproof nonstick pan over medium heat. Add the onion and cook until soft, about 5 minutes. Stir in the garlic, then add the zucchini. Cook until the zucchini has softened and the onions have turned golden brown, about 8 minutes. Season with 1 teaspoon of the salt.

3. Stir in the red peppers and baby spinach, allowing the spinach to wilt.

4. In a medium bowl, whisk the eggs, herbs, cheese, remaining ½ teaspoon salt, and black pepper until combined.

5. Pour the egg mixture into the pan and use a spatula to stir the mixture together. Cook for a bit, then run the spatula around the edge and gently shake and tilt the pan as necessary to allow the uncooked egg to run underneath. Reduce the heat to low, cover, and cook for 5 to 7 minutes, until the egg is almost set.

6. Remove the lid and place the pan under the broiler for 1 to 2 minutes, until the top is golden brown. Remove from the heat and shake the pan to ensure the egg isn't sticking; use a spatula to gently lift the sides if so. Carefully slide the frittata onto a platter and cut into wedges. Serve immediately.

Soft Herb and Mushroom Omelet

Serves: 1

Prep Time: 5 minutes

Cook Time: 10 minutes

1 cup sliced cremini mushrooms

2 tablespoons grass-fed unsalted butter

1 garlic clove, minced

3 large pasture-raised organic eggs

1 tablespoon finely chopped fresh tarragon leaves

½ teaspoon kosher salt

¼ teaspoon freshly ground black pepper

For a quick and versatile breakfast, an omelet is about as simple as it gets. Eggs are one of the easiest, most healthful ingredients: Loaded with protein, vitamins, and minerals like biotin, which can keep our skin strong and elastic, they provide many anti-aging benefits. Once you've mastered the technique of making an omelet, the flavor combinations are endless. I love using hearty mushrooms, which are low in calories and high in B vitamins and have a meaty texture and umami flavor. This savory omelet is ideal for breakfast but would also be great for a light dinner paired with a crisp green salad.

1. Heat an 8-inch nonstick pan over medium heat. Add the sliced mushrooms and cook, stirring occasionally, until they begin to soften and sweat, about 3 minutes. Add 1 tablespoon of the butter and the garlic and continue cooking for 3 minutes, until they take on color. Remove the mushrooms from the pan and set aside.

2. In a small bowl, whisk the eggs, tarragon, salt, and pepper. In the same pan used for the mushrooms, melt the remaining 1 tablespoon butter over medium heat until it begins to bubble. Add the eggs, tilting the pan to evenly distribute them. Cook, using a spatula to gently scrape the eggs toward the center and tilting the pan to allow the uncooked egg to run underneath, for a few minutes.

3. Reduce the heat to low and scatter the mushrooms on one side of the omelet. As soon as the eggs are set on the bottom but still slightly runny on top, gently jerk the pan towards you to loosen the eggs. Use your spatula to carefully fold the bare half of the omelet over the mushrooms. Tilt the omelet onto a plate and serve immediately.

Tex-Mex Breakfast Bake

Serves: 6 to 8

Prep Time: 20 minutes

Cook Time: 1 hour

2 tablespoons avocado oil

¾ pound turkey sausage, casings removed

2 medium sweet potatoes, peeled and cubed

1 yellow onion, chopped

1 bunch scallions, white and light green parts sliced, greens thinly sliced and reserved for garnish

1 red bell pepper, stemmed, seeded, and chopped

1 jalapeño pepper, stemmed, seeded, and finely chopped (optional)

2 garlic cloves, minced

2 teaspoons smoked paprika

1 teaspoon ground cumin

1 teaspoon chili powder

1½ teaspoons kosher salt

1 small bunch green or Tuscan kale, deveined and roughly chopped

12 large pasture-raised organic eggs

½ cup nondairy milk

½ teaspoon freshly ground black pepper

Sometimes you need a brunch dish that can easily feed a crowd. This large-scale frittata is just that, a flavorful blend of eggs and sausage, kale, sweet potatoes, and warm spices. You can make the sausage and potato mixture ahead of time and refrigerate; however, you may need to adjust the cooking time slightly.

1. Preheat the oven to 325°F. Lightly grease a 9x13-inch casserole dish.

2. Heat the avocado oil in a large frying pan over medium heat. Add the sausage meat and cook, breaking the meat up with a wooden spoon into smaller pieces, until golden brown, about 5 minutes.

3. To the same pan, add the sweet potatoes and cook for 5 to 7 minutes, until fork tender. Add the onion and white and light green parts of the scallions, stirring well until they have softened, about 3 minutes. Add the bell pepper, jalapeño (if using), garlic, paprika, cumin, chili powder, and 1 teaspoon of the salt. Stir the mixture together, then turn off the heat and stir in the kale. Transfer the mixture to the prepared casserole dish and let cool slightly.

4. In a large bowl, whisk together the eggs and milk and season with the remaining ½ teaspoon salt and the pepper. Pour the eggs into the prepared baking dish, using a spoon to mix everything together. Bake until the casserole is golden brown and firm to the touch, about 35 minutes. Let stand for 10 minutes, sprinkle with scallion greens, and serve.

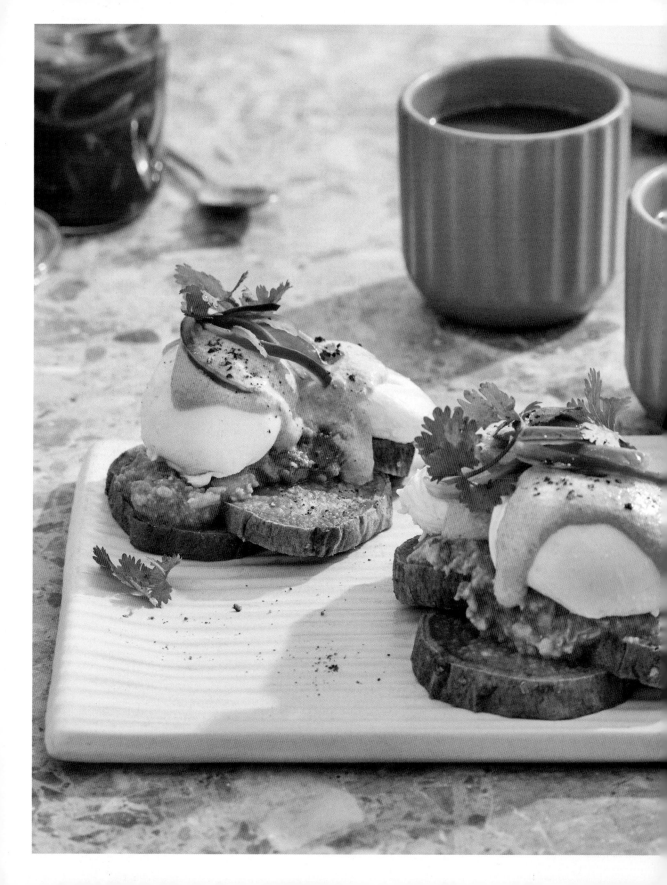

Sweet Potato and Egg Stacks

Serves: 4

Prep Time: 15 minutes

Cook Time: 30 minutes

Sweet Potatoes

2 medium sweet potatoes, scrubbed clean and sliced into ½-inch-thick rounds

2 tablespoons extra-virgin olive oil

1 teaspoon ground cumin

½ teaspoon kosher salt

Avocado Mash

1 ripe medium avocado, halved, pitted, and peeled

Grated zest and juice of 1 lime

1 tablespoon finely chopped fresh cilantro leaves, plus more for garnish

½ teaspoon kosher salt

Poached Eggs

1 tablespoon distilled vinegar

8 large pasture-raised organic eggs

To Serve

1 cup Cashew Hollandaise (page 204), gently warmed

½ cup Pickled Red Onions (page 210)

Freshly ground black pepper

A twist on classic eggs Benedict, I've swapped out the English muffin for more nutritious roasted sweet potatoes. Antioxidant-rich avocado provides an extra dose of anti-aging benefits from their inflammation-fighting fatty acids and vitamins that protect our skin. Topped with a cashew-based vegan hollandaise, this dish will remain the decadent star of your brunch.

1. Preheat the oven to 400°F. Line a baking sheet with parchment paper.

2. **For the potatoes:** In a large bowl combine the sweet potatoes, olive oil, cumin, and salt. Arrange in a single layer on the lined baking sheet. Roast for 20 minutes, flipping halfway, until softened.

3. **For the avocado mash:** In a small bowl, use a fork to mash the avocado with the lime zest, juice, and cilantro. Stir in the salt.

4. **For the eggs:** Bring a deep pot or saucepan of water to a boil over high heat. Add the vinegar and reduce to a simmer. Crack the eggs into teacups or small bowls. Gently but quickly, add the eggs to the simmering water. Poach for 4 to 5 minutes, until the whites have set completely. Use a slotted spoon to transfer the eggs to a paper towel–lined plate.

5. To serve, stack two or three rounds of sweet potato on each plate. Top with a spoonful of mashed avocado and two poached eggs. Drizzle with the hollandaise and garnish with additional cilantro, pickled onions, and a good crack of black pepper.

Tempeh Sausage with Eggs and Roasted Tomatoes

Serves: 4

Prep Time: 30 minutes, including chilling time

Cook Time: 1 hour

Tempeh patties are a great plan-ahead meal because they keep well in the fridge for a couple of days. Packed with nutritious mushrooms and easily digestible tempeh, the protein-packed patties are a delicious plant-based alternative to your traditional breakfast sausage.

Roasted Tomatoes

6 plum tomatoes, halved lengthwise

2 tablespoons extra-virgin olive oil

1 garlic clove, thinly sliced

Leaves from 2 sprigs fresh thyme, plus extra for garnish

Tempeh Patties

8 ounces tempeh

2 tablespoons avocado oil

½ small yellow onion, roughly chopped

1 garlic clove, minced

1 cup roughly chopped cremini mushrooms

2 teaspoons thyme leaves

1 teaspoon paprika

½ teaspoon red pepper flakes

1 teaspoon kosher salt

½ teaspoon freshly ground black pepper

Poached Eggs

1 tablespoon vinegar

4 large pasture-raised organic eggs

To Serve

2 cups baby spinach

Kosher salt and freshly ground black pepper, to taste

1. **For the tomatoes:** Preheat the oven to 350°F. Place the tomato halves in a baking dish cut side up, drizzle with the olive oil, and sprinkle on the garlic and thyme. Roast for 30 to 40 minutes, until softened and caramelized. Set aside. Leave the oven on.

2. **For the tempeh patties:** Bring a pot of water to a boil over high heat. Add the tempeh and cook for 10 minutes, until soft. Transfer to a paper towel–lined plate to drain. (This helps to remove the bitter taste and soften the tempeh for the patties.)

3. Heat 1 tablespoon of the avocado oil in a pan over medium heat. Add the onion and sauté until translucent, 4 to 6 minutes. Add the garlic and continue to cook for 1 minute. Add the mushrooms and cook for about 8 minutes, until the pan is dry. Stir in the thyme, paprika, and red pepper flakes. Season with the salt and pepper.

4. Transfer the mushroom mixture to a food processor and pulse until it begins to resemble a crumble. Add the boiled tempeh and continue pulsing until the mixture sticks together when pressed between your hands. Divide the mixture into four portions and gently flatten. Refrigerate for at least 10 minutes. The patties can be made up to 2 days ahead and kept in the refrigerator.

5. Line a baking sheet with parchment paper. Heat a nonstick skillet over medium heat. Add the remaining 1 tablespoon avocado oil to the pan and gently cook the tempeh patties for 3 minutes on each side. Transfer to the baking sheet and bake for 5 minutes, until golden brown.

6. **Meanwhile, for the eggs:** Bring a deep pot or saucepan of water to a boil over high heat. Add the vinegar and reduce to a simmer. Crack the eggs into teacups or small bowls, then gently but quickly add the eggs to the simmering water. Poach for 4 to 5 minutes, until the whites have set completely. Use a slotted spoon to transfer the eggs to a paper towel–lined plate to drain.

7. Divide the spinach among four plates. Top with a tempeh patty, poached egg, and tomatoes. Sprinkle with additional thyme and a pinch of salt and pepper.

Baked Eggs with Chickpeas and Tomatoes

Serves: 2 to 4

Prep Time: 10 minutes

Cook Time: 35 minutes

Baked Eggs

2 tablespoons extra-virgin olive oil

4 garlic cloves, smashed

½ teaspoon red pepper flakes

1 (28-ounce) can San Marzano or other good-quality tomatoes

½ teaspoon kosher salt, plus more to taste

¼ teaspoon freshly ground black pepper

1 (15.5-ounce) can chickpeas, drained and rinsed

6 large pasture-raised organic eggs

Herb Salad

2 cups mixed fresh soft herbs, such as watercress, parsley, and cilantro

1 shallot, sliced

2 tablespoons extra-virgin olive oil

1 tablespoon lemon juice

1½ teaspoons red wine vinegar

Pinch of kosher salt

Slow-cooked eggs in a garlicky tomato sauce is a delicious one-pan meal. Cooked tomatoes contain lycopene, a phytonutrient that helps support cognitive and heart health. I've pumped up the protein and fiber with chickpeas, making it a hearty option for breakfast, lunch, or dinner.

1. Heat the olive oil in a large skillet fitted with a lid over medium heat. Add the garlic and red pepper flakes and cook, stirring, until the garlic begins to turn golden, about 1 minute. Add the tomatoes and salt and use a fork or wooden spoon to break up the tomatoes. Reduce the heat to low and cook, stirring often, for 15 to 20 minutes, until the sauce has begun to thicken and no longer runs together when a spoon is dragged through. Season with salt and pepper, then add the chickpeas. Stir, cover, and continue cooking for another 10 minutes.

2. Use the back of a spoon to create six 2-inch-wide indentations in the sauce. Gently crack an egg into each indentation. Cover the pan and cook for 4 to 5 minutes, until the whites set.

3. For the herb salad: While the eggs are cooking, mix the herbs in a large bowl with the shallot, olive oil, lemon juice, and vinegar. Season with salt.

4. Scoop the cooked eggs and chickpeas into shallow bowls and top with the herb salad.

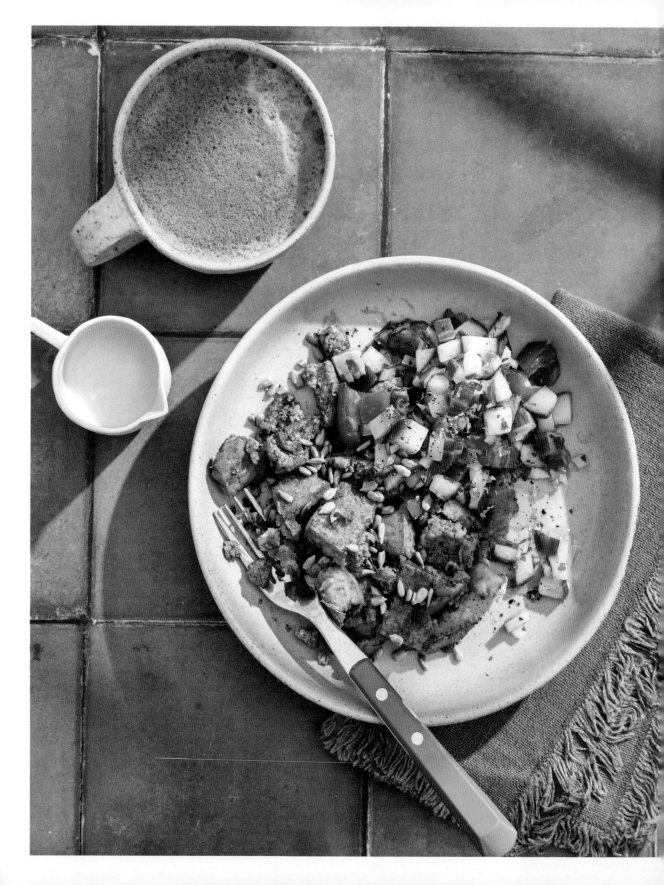

Smoky Scrambled Tofu with Chopped Salad

Serves: 4

Prep Time: 20 minutes

Cook Time: 10 minutes

Tofu

1 (12-ounce) block extra-firm organic tofu

¼ cup water

2 tablespoons coconut aminos or gluten-free tamari

1 garlic clove, grated

½ teaspoon smoked paprika

½ teaspoon ground cumin

½ teaspoon ground turmeric

½ teaspoon kosher salt

1 tablespoon avocado oil

½ cup finely chopped white onion

Salad

¼ cup finely chopped white onion

1 large tomato, diced

¼ English cucumber, quartered and diced

2 tablespoons finely chopped fresh flat-leaf parsley

1 teaspoon grated lemon zest

2 tablespoons lemon juice

1 tablespoon extra-virgin olive oil

¼ teaspoon kosher salt, plus more to taste

¼ cup toasted sunflower seeds, for garnish

This quick tofu scramble will convert even egg-loving skeptics. Tofu is a healthy plant-based alternative that's packed with protein and amino acids to support overall health and contains essential vitamins and minerals like calcium and vitamin A, which keep our bones strong. Paired perfectly with a bright chopped salad, this flavorful breakfast is sure to keep you satisfied throughout your morning.

1. **For the tofu:** Begin by slicing the tofu into 4½-inch-thick strips. Press the tofu between sheets of paper towel by placing a heavy skillet on top for about 15 minutes; this helps to remove the excess moisture. This step can be done ahead up to 1 hour. Set aside while you prepare the salad.

2. **For the salad:** In a large bowl combine the onion, tomato, cucumber, and parsley. Stir, then add the lemon zest, juice, and olive oil. Season with salt.

3. In a small bowl, make the tofu sauce by mixing the water, coconut aminos, garlic, paprika, cumin, turmeric, and salt.

4. Heat the avocado oil in a skillet over medium heat. Add the tofu strips and cook for 4 minutes, until golden and crisp. Flip the blocks and continue cooking for another 3 minutes. Lower the heat and add the onion, using a wooden spoon to break up the tofu into smaller chunks. Mix the onion through for about 3 minutes, until it has softened. Season with a pinch of salt. Add the tofu sauce and continue stirring and breaking up the tofu, until all the liquid is absorbed.

5. Serve immediately with a scoop of the chopped salad and a sprinkle of sunflower seeds.

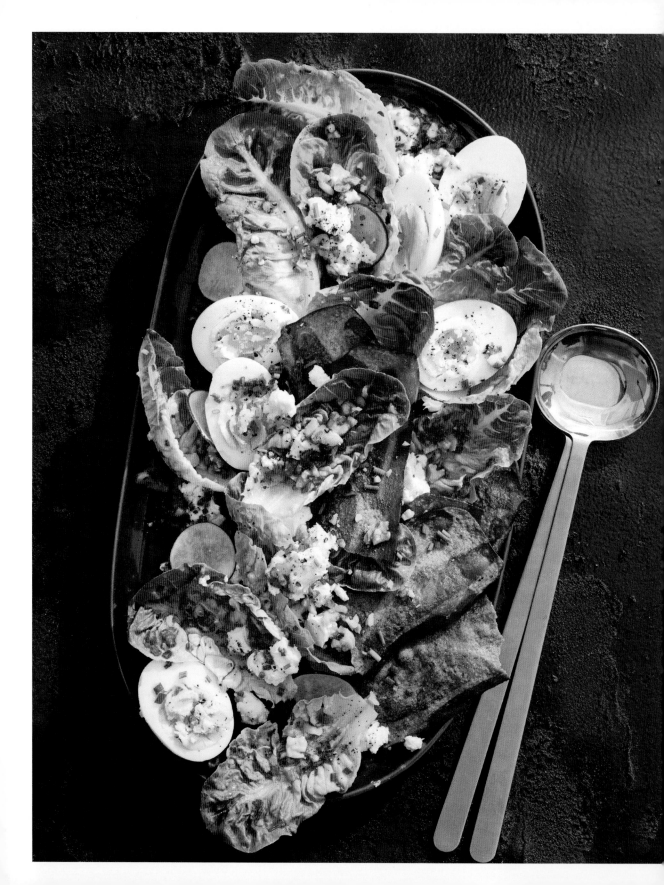

Savory Breakfast Salad

Serves: 4

Prep Time: 15 minutes

Cook Time: 25 minutes

Breakfast Salad

4 slices turkey bacon

4 large pasture-raised organic eggs

4 heads Little Gem lettuce, leaves separated

4 large radishes, thinly sliced

1 cup leftover cooked grains, such as quinoa or brown rice (optional)

4 ounces soft goat cheese, crumbled

Dressing

¼ cup extra-virgin olive oil

1 tablespoon fresh lemon juice

1 tablespoon apple cider vinegar

1 teaspoon Dijon mustard

2 tablespoons finely chopped fresh chives

½ teaspoon kosher salt

¼ teaspoon freshly ground black pepper

½ cup finely chopped toasted walnut pieces

Salad for breakfast? It may not seem like your typical choice, but this salad—packed with crunchy greens, protein-rich cheese, heart-healthy eggs, and lean turkey bacon—is a great start to your day, and the protein-packed ingredients are essential for healthy aging. I love adding a scoop of leftover grains from the fridge, but it's equally as wholesome without.

1. **For the breakfast salad:** Preheat the oven to 400°F. Line a baking sheet with parchment paper, then a wire rack. Arrange the turkey bacon on the rack and bake for 10 minutes. Flip the strips and continue baking for another 5 minutes, until crisp.

2. Meanwhile, bring a pot of water to a boil over high heat. Using a spoon, gently lower the eggs into the water and cook for 8 minutes. Transfer the eggs with a slotted spoon to a bowl of ice water. Once cool, peel the eggs, halve, and set aside.

3. **For the dressing:** Combine all the ingredients except the walnuts in a bowl, stirring to emulsify. Stir in the walnuts and taste; adjust the seasoning if necessary.

4. In a large bowl, combine the lettuce, radishes, grains (if using), and a couple tablespoons of the dressing, mixing well. Divide the salad among four bowls and top with the turkey bacon, goat cheese, and egg halves. Drizzle with remaining dressing and serve.

Protein Powerhouse Smoothie

Serves: 1

Prep Time: 5 minutes

1 cup macadamia nut milk
(or milk of choice)

1 cup frozen wild blueberries
(or fresh blueberries, see Tip)

1 scoop whey or vegan protein
powder

2 teaspoons ground flaxseed

1 tablespoon almond butter
(or other nut butter of choice)

1 tablespoon chia seeds

1 teaspoon ground cinnamon

1 teaspoon maple syrup
(optional)

This creamy and nutty smoothie is a perfect protein-packed addition to your morning routine. Chia seeds are one of the best plant proteins out there. They contain all nine essential amino acids and are a good source of fiber in just one small serving. Fresh blueberries are a superfood, and if you can find wild blueberries, they are an even greater source of antioxidants and vitamins that help support cognitive and mental health. I love to use macadamia nut milk for its delicious flavor and creaminess, but you can substitute any dairy-free milk.

Add all the ingredients to a blender and blend until smooth, about 1 minute.

Tip: *If you don't have frozen blueberries on hand, add 1 cup of ice along with fresh blueberries and blend.*

Antioxidant Berry Smoothie

Serves: 1 to 2

Prep Time: 10 minutes

¾ cup pomegranate juice

1 small beet, peeled and
roughly chopped

½ cup fresh or frozen
blackberries

1 (1-inch) piece fresh ginger,
peeled

2 tablespoons lemon juice

1 scoop protein powder

I love this earthy blend of beet, pomegranate, and blackberry. Slightly creamier than a cold-pressed juice, the smoothie is packed with powerful antioxidants. Pomegranates are loaded with polyphenolic compounds that protect your cells from free radicals. They also contain a unique compound called punicalagin, which helps preserve the collagen in your skin; beets are one of the richest sources of glutamine, a gut-friendly amino acid.

Add all the ingredients to a blender with 1 cup of ice and blend until smooth, about 1 minute.

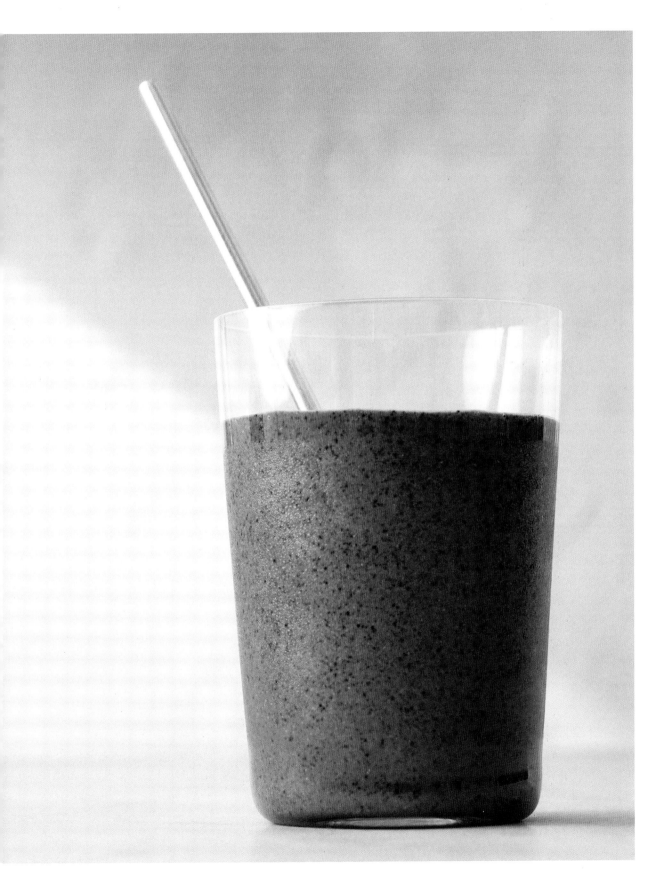

Ultimate Recovery Smoothie

Serves: 2
Prep Time: 15 minutes

¼ cup raw cashews

Boiling water

1 pitted Medjool date

1 banana, frozen

1 cup cold brewed coffee

¼ cup unsweetened almond milk
(or milk of choice)

1 tablespoon MCT oil

1 tablespoon cashew butter

1 tablespoon chia seeds

1 teaspoon ground cinnamon

For those mornings when you need that extra boost of caffeine, use leftover cold coffee to make this better-than-a-Frappuccino blend. Laced with warm cinnamon and creamy cashew butter and boosted with MCT oil, which contains anti-inflammatory lauric acid that is helpful for healthy skin, this coffee-based smoothie is a sure bet to get your day started on the right foot.

1. Place the cashews and date into a heatproof bowl, cover with just boiled water, and let soak for 5 minutes. Drain.

2. Add the remaining ingredients and 1 cup ice to a blender. Add the drained nuts and date and blend until smooth and thick, about 1 minute.

Super-Matcha Smoothie

Serves: 1

Prep Time: 10 minutes

1 cup macadamia nut milk
(or milk of choice)

1 cup spinach leaves

¾ cup frozen mango

1 scoop protein powder

½ teaspoon matcha powder

1 tablespoon cashew butter

Pinch ground cardamom
(optional)

Matcha is a powerful green tea known for its cancer-fighting, high-antioxidant compounds and overall health benefits. Although it contains caffeine, it won't leave you feeling jittery due to a very special amino acid called L-theanine, a biologically active compound that helps reduce stress and boosts the body's defense enzymes. Matcha pairs well with tropical flavors, like the mango in this smoothie.

Add all the ingredients to a blender and blend until smooth, about 1 minute.

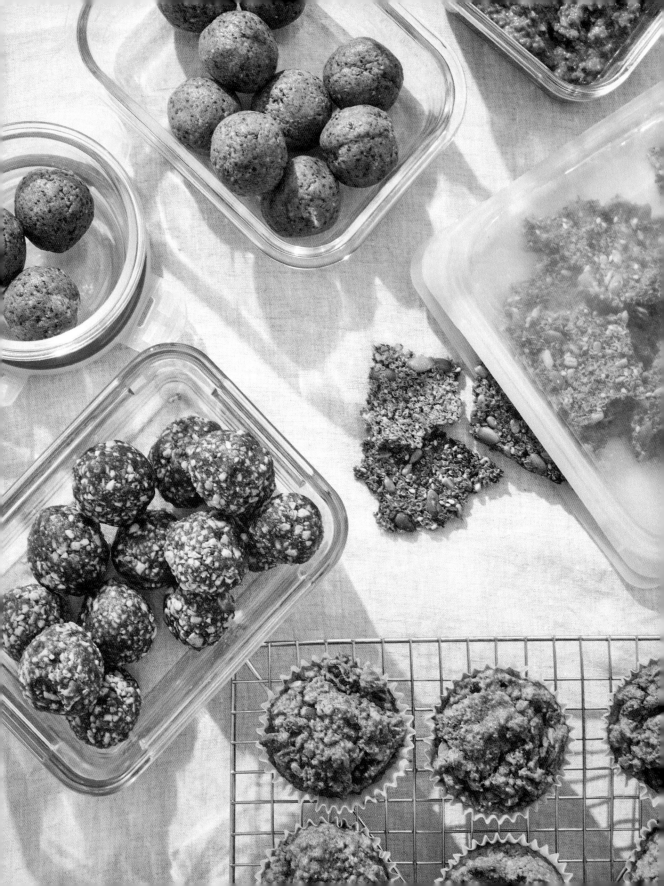

Snacks

Everyone loves a good snack, especially when it satisfies a craving and fills the void between meals. The retail snack category is one of the fastest growing, but store-bought snacks are filled with hidden sugars and additives that aren't beneficial to your health. Consuming high-fiber, high-protein snacks between meals can keep your blood sugar stable and provide essential vitamins and antioxidants helpful in the anti-aging process. So it's worth putting in the time to make your own snacks and controlling the amount of salt, sugar, and flavor that goes into them. My favorites of the bunch are my spiced Ginger and Cashew Energy Balls (page 29), Paleo Trail-Mix Muffins (page 34), and savory Mushroom Tapenade (page 41). All of these treats can be made ahead of time, and most can be batch-prepared, with the goal to get you eating healthy and well day to day.

Goji and Coconut Trail Mix

Makes: 6 cups
Prep Time: 5 minutes
Cook Time: 10 minutes

1 cup raw cashews

1 cup raw whole almonds

1 cup raw Brazil nuts

1 cup raw pumpkin seeds

1 teaspoon ground cinnamon

1 tablespoon coconut oil, melted

2 tablespoons maple syrup

1 cup goji berries

½ teaspoon flaky sea salt

½ cup dark (70 percent cacao) chocolate chips (optional)

Homemade trail mix is a delicious on-the-go snack. This easily adaptable recipe is perfect post-workout, on a hike, or midday at work. It contains antioxidants, healthy fats, protein, and iron, helping stave off cravings and keep you feeling fuller longer. Nuts are full of powerful anti-aging nutrients that help reduce your risk of age-related disease such as heart disease and diabetes.

1. Preheat the oven to 350°F. Line a baking sheet with parchment paper.

2. In a large bowl, combine the cashews, almonds, Brazil nuts, and pumpkin seeds. Sprinkle with the cinnamon, melted coconut oil, and maple syrup and mix well. Transfer to the baking sheet and roast for 10 minutes, until lightly golden. Let cool completely.

3. Stir in the goji berries, sea salt, and chocolate, if using.

4. Store in an airtight container in the fridge for up to 2 months.

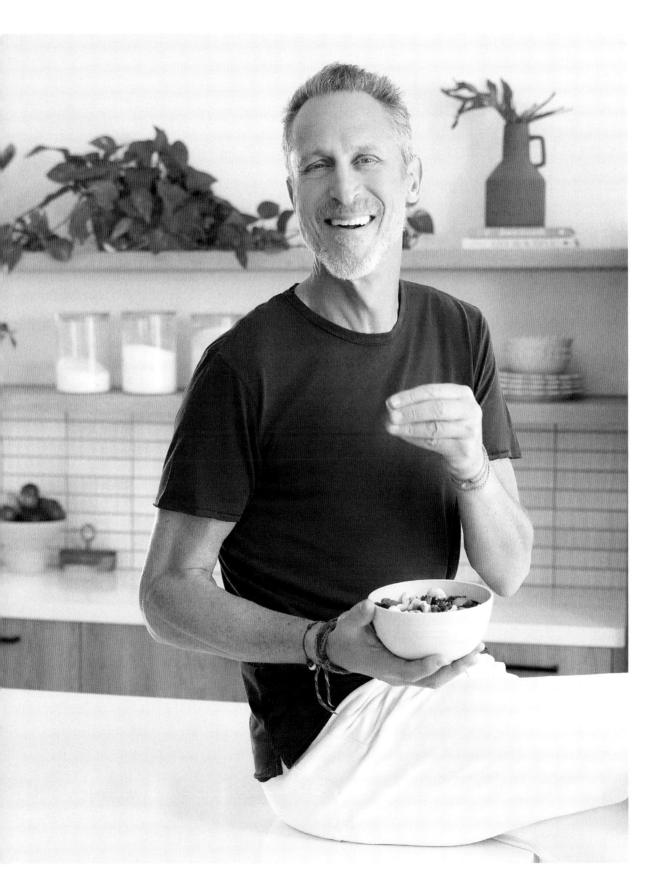

Nut Butter Protein Balls

Makes: 13 balls

Prep Time: 10 minutes

⅔ cup peanut butter
(or other nut/seed butter)

½ cup hulled hemp seeds

5 tablespoons unflavored whey
or plant-based protein powder

2 tablespoons chia seeds

1 tablespoon maple syrup

1 ½ teaspoons ground cinnamon

1 teaspoon vanilla extract

I absolutely love these energy bites because of their versatility and high protein content. Your body needs protein to function throughout the day, helping to build muscle and produce the hormones and enzymes required to keep you healthy. These balls are packed with so many of the highly nutritious ingredients that keep you feeling full longer: Chia seeds provide a healthy dose of fiber and protein, while hemp seeds and protein powder add an additional boost of protein and vitamins. These are a great snack post-workout, and they keep well when refrigerated. You can easily substitute another nut or seed butter if you are sensitive to allergens.

1. In a food processor, combine all the ingredients. Blend until the mixture comes together when pressed between your fingers. Roll into about thirteen golf ball–sized balls.

2. Store in an airtight container in the fridge for up to 2 months.

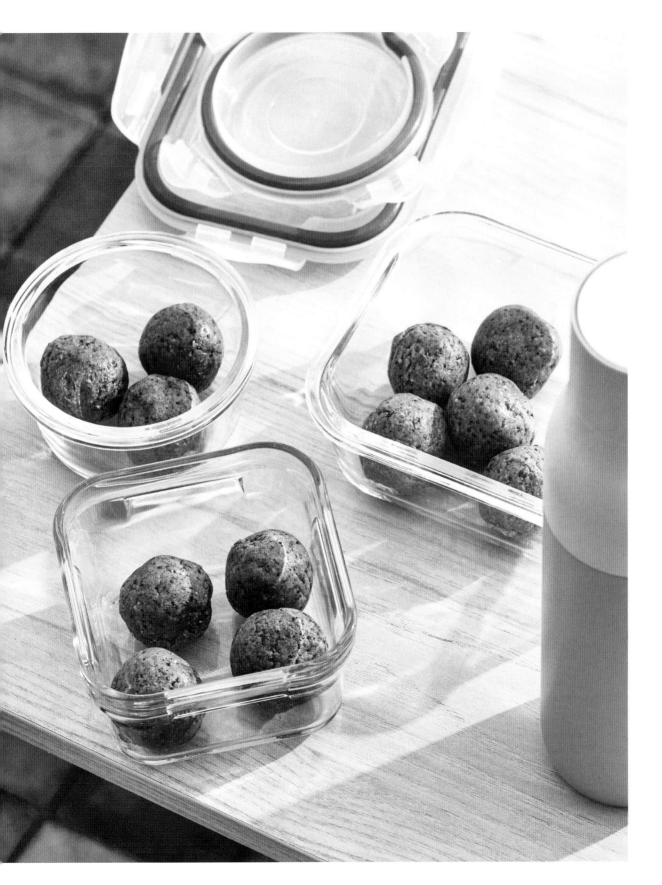

Spicy Edamame Hummus

Makes: 2 cups

Prep Time: 10 minutes

1 cup frozen edamame, defrosted

1 (15.5-ounce) can chickpeas, drained and rinsed

1 to 2 jalapeño peppers, seeded and roughly chopped

¼ cup unsweetened dairy-free milk

⅓ cup lemon or lime juice

1 tablespoon almond butter

1 tablespoon extra-virgin olive oil

1½ teaspoons kosher salt

1 cup loosely packed fresh cilantro leaves

This edamame dip is a twist on traditional chickpea hummus. Edamame are an excellent source of phytoestrogens, compounds that have been linked to a reduced risk of heart disease and poor bone health. Loaded with protein from both the chickpeas and edamame and packed with bright, fresh flavors, it's a delicious dip or spread to serve with veggies, Super-Seed Quinoa Crackers (page 33), or simple grilled chicken.

1. In a blender or food processor, combine the edamame, chickpeas, and jalapeños and blend until chopped. Add the milk, citrus juice, almond butter, olive oil, salt, and cilantro. Blend until very smooth and creamy, about 2 minutes.

2. Store in an airtight container in the refrigerator for up to 1 week.

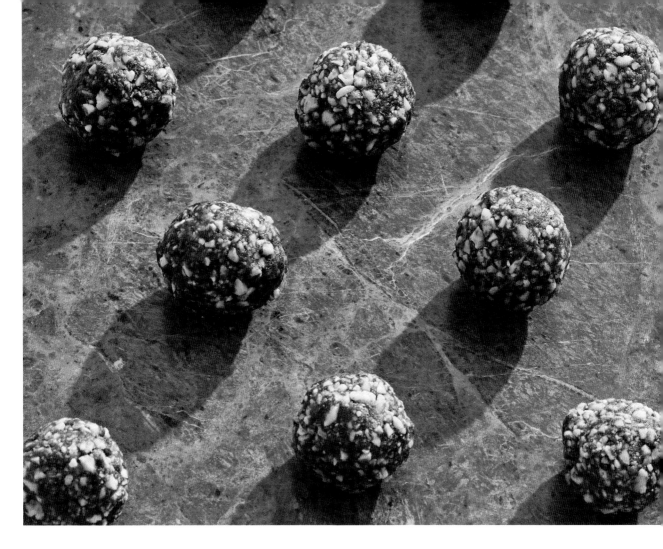

Ginger and Cashew Energy Balls

Makes: 18 balls

Prep Time: 10 minutes

2 cups raw cashews

1 teaspoon ground ginger

½ teaspoon ground cinnamon

½ cup (6 to 7) pitted Medjool dates

¼ cup almond butter

1 to 2 tablespoons blackstrap molasses

These energy bites taste like ginger snap cookies, except they're more nutritious! Cashews provide a good source of healthy fats and protein, which can lower your cholesterol, while the blackstrap molasses gives you a significant amount of your daily iron.

1.   In a food processor, combine the cashews, ginger, and cinnamon. Pulse a few times, until the mixture is crumbly. Add the dates, almond butter, and 1 tablespoon molasses and continue pulsing until the mixture comes together and sticks when pressed between your fingers; add more molasses if needed. Roll the mixture into about eighteen golf ball–sized bites.

2.   Store in an airtight container in the fridge for up to 2 months.

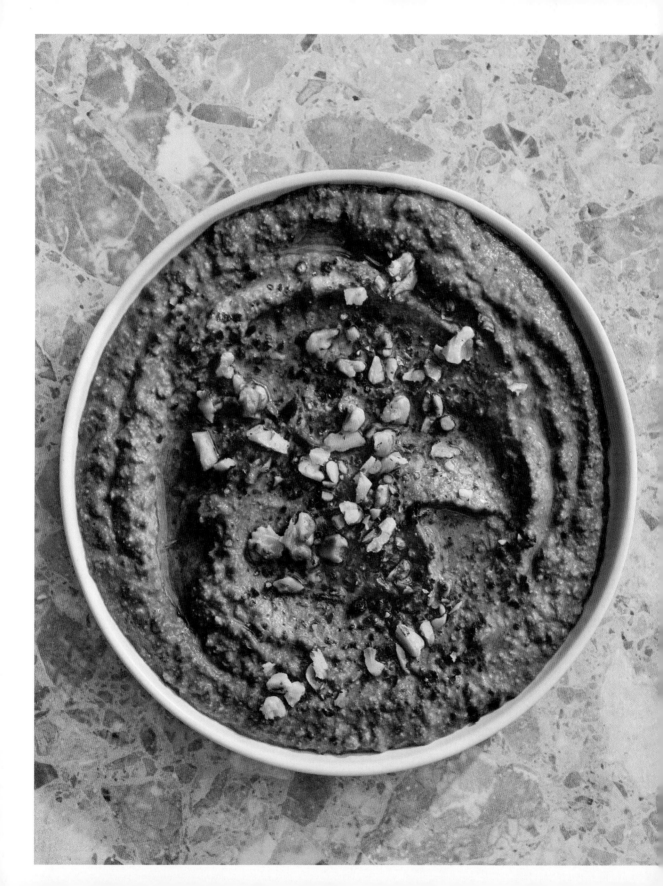

Smoky Roasted Pepper and Walnut Dip

Makes: 1½ cups

Prep Time: 15 minutes

1 cup roasted red peppers from a jar, drained

½ cup toasted walnut pieces, plus more for garnish

2 tablespoons almond flour

½ teaspoon toasted cumin seeds

2 tablespoons extra-virgin olive oil, plus more for serving

2 tablespoons fresh lemon juice

1 tablespoon pomegranate molasses

1 tablespoon tomato puree

1 teaspoon Aleppo pepper flakes

1 teaspoon smoked paprika

1 teaspoon kosher salt, or to taste

I can't get enough of this vibrant red pepper dip. Seasoned with just enough spice and a touch of sweetness, it's the perfect snack. Rich in omega-3 fatty acids from the walnuts, which can improve your energy and keep your heart healthy, the dip is full of other nutrients—and flavor. Bonus: You can whip it up in no time. Serve with veggies or gluten-free seed crackers, such as Super-Seed Quinoa Crackers (page 33).

1. In a food processor, combine the red peppers, walnuts, almond flour, and cumin. Pulse a few times until the mixture is slightly blended. Add the olive oil, lemon juice, pomegranate molasses, tomato puree, Aleppo pepper, and paprika. Blend until smooth, then season with the salt.

2. Transfer the dip to a bowl. Using the back of a spoon, smooth the top, then create swirls. Top with a drizzle of olive oil and the remaining chopped walnut pieces.

3. Store in an airtight container in the refrigerator for up to 1 week.

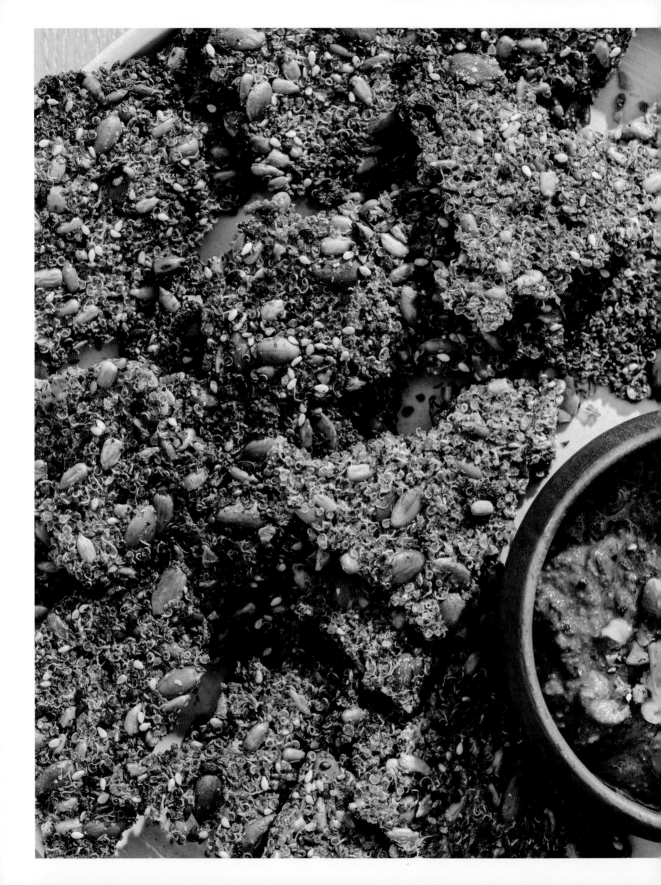

Super-Seed Quinoa Crackers

Makes: 20 to 30 crackers
Prep Time: 25 minutes
Cook Time: 45 minutes

1½ cups cooked quinoa

⅓ cup raw pumpkin seeds

⅓ cup raw sunflower seeds

¼ cup ground flaxseed

1 tablespoon chia seeds

1 cup boiling water

1 tablespoon sesame seeds

1 tablespoon black sesame seeds

1 tablespoon garlic powder

1 tablespoon dried onion flakes

½ teaspoon flaky sea salt

Homemade crackers may sound daunting, but these are incredibly easy and worth the effort. Quinoa is a powerful plant protein. Although classified as a whole grain, it is actually an edible seed that contains all nine amino acids, is filled with fiber, and is gluten-free. Blended with flaxseed, chia, sesame, and pumpkin seeds, then topped with everything bagel seasonings, the crackers are irresistible as soon as they come out of the oven!

1. In a large heatproof bowl, combine the quinoa, pumpkin seeds, sunflower seeds, flaxseed, and chia seeds. Pour the boiling water over the mixture and let sit for 20 minutes.

2. Meanwhile, in a small bowl, combine the sesame seeds, black sesame seeds, garlic powder, onion flakes, and sea salt.

3. Preheat the oven to 350°F. Line a standard 13x18-inch baking sheet with parchment paper.

4. Transfer the quinoa mixture to the prepared baking sheet and use a spatula to spread it as thin and even as possible, to all edges of the sheet. Sprinkle the seasonings all over. Bake for 45 minutes, turning the baking sheet halfway, until golden brown. Let cool completely before breaking with your hands into large crackers.

5. Store in an airtight container for up to 2 weeks.

Paleo Trail-Mix Muffins

Makes: 12 muffins

Prep Time: 10 minutes

Cook Time: 30 minutes

1 large apple, cored

1 large carrot, peeled

2 large pasture-raised organic eggs

¼ cup extra-virgin olive oil

2 tablespoons maple syrup

2 cups almond flour

1 teaspoon baking soda

½ teaspoon baking powder

2 tablespoons ground flaxseed

1 teaspoon ground cinnamon

¼ teaspoon kosher salt

⅓ cup raw pumpkin seeds

⅓ cup raw sunflower seeds

⅓ cup dried cherries or cranberries

These muffins are one of my go-to snacks. Naturally gluten-free and high in fiber and protein, they are the perfect healthy snack for noshing between meals. They are also easy to make, with everything tossed into the food processor, which then does the work for you.

1. Preheat the oven to 350°F. Line a standard 12-cup muffin tin with paper liners.

2. In a food processor fitted with the grater attachment (or with a box grater), grate the apple and carrot.

3. Switch out the grater attachment for the standard food processor blade. Add the eggs to the carrot and apple and pulse a few times, until the mixture comes together.

4. Add the olive oil, maple syrup, almond flour, baking soda, baking powder, flaxseed, cinnamon, and salt. Blend until the mixture is almost smooth. With a spatula, gently stir in the pumpkin seeds, sunflower seeds, and dried fruit until combined.

5. Using an ice cream scoop or large spoon, evenly scoop the mixture into the prepared muffin cups. Bake for 25 to 28 minutes, until the muffins are puffed and golden. Allow to cool completely before serving.

6. Store in an airtight container in the refrigerator for up to 1 week.

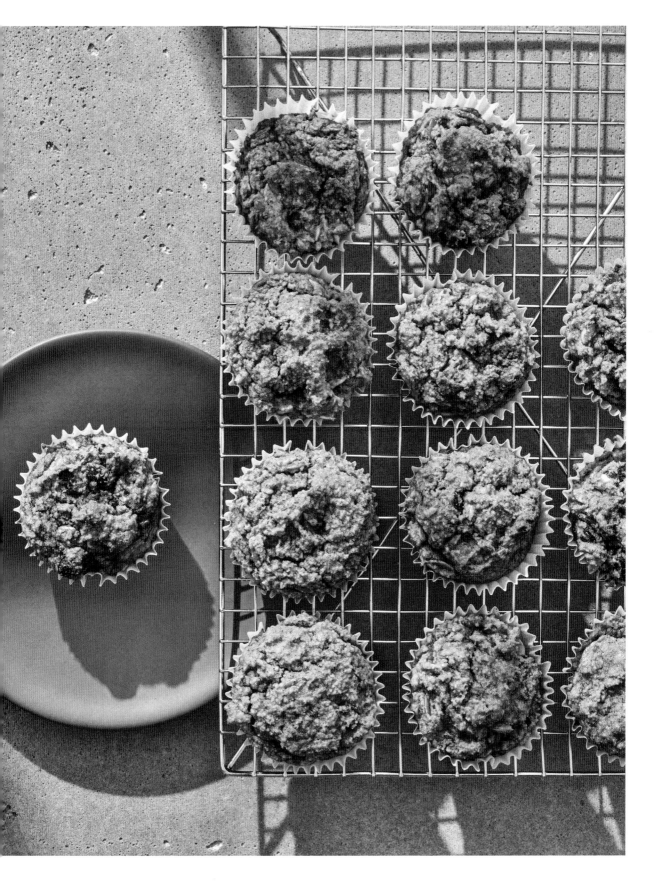

Oven-Baked Miso Kale Chips

Makes: 4 cups

Prep Time: 5 minutes

Cook Time: 35 minutes

1 teaspoon avocado oil

1 teaspoon white miso paste

1 teaspoon maple syrup

½ teaspoon gluten-free tamari

1 large bunch green or Tuscan kale, deveined and torn into large pieces

2 tablespoons toasted sesame seeds

This is a great way to use up any leftover or sad-looking kale that's spent a bit too much time in your fridge drawer: Roasting the leaves at a low temperature allows them to crisp up nicely. Kale is a delicious dark leafy green high in vitamin C and selenium, which can help support a healthy immune system. Coated with miso, a fermented soybean paste that contains probiotics linked to a healthier gut microbiome and reduced blood pressure, these crispy kale chips are a healthy and tasty snack.

1. Preheat the oven to 300°F. Line one or two baking sheets (depending how much kale you have) with parchment paper.

2. In a large bowl, mix the avocado oil, miso, maple syrup, and tamari. Add the kale leaves and use your hands to massage the oil mixture into the leaves, ensuring they are well covered.

3. Transfer the kale to the baking sheets, making sure to not overcrowd the leaves (otherwise they won't crisp up). Bake for 30 minutes, rotating the baking sheets halfway, until crisp. Turn the oven off and leave the sheets inside for another 5 minutes before removing. Allow to cool, then sprinkle with the sesame seeds.

4. Store in an airtight container for up to 5 days.

Tomato and Sardine Crisps

Serves: 2 to 4

Prep Time: 20 minutes

1 tomato, finely chopped

½ cup finely diced avocado

¼ cup finely minced red onion

1 tablespoon extra-virgin olive oil

1 tablespoon lemon juice

½ teaspoon kosher salt

1 (4-ounce) can wild-caught boneless sardines, drained

2 tablespoons finely chopped dill

Freshly ground black pepper, to taste

Gluten-free crackers, for serving

This is a great spread to make when you're looking for a quick snack or light lunch, or even entertaining friends. Sardines are often overlooked at the supermarket, but they are inexpensive, shelf-stable, readily available, and an excellent source of omega-3 fatty acids, vitamin D, and calcium. They are also low in mercury, making them a healthy canned fish alternative.

1. In a bowl, mix the tomato, avocado, and onion. Stir in the olive oil and lemon juice and season with the salt. Add the sardines, gently breaking them up with a fork. Gently stir in the dill and season to taste with black pepper.

2. Using a spoon, scoop the mixture onto crackers and serve.

3. Store any remaining sardine spread in an airtight container in the refrigerator for up to 2 days.

Egg Snack Pots, Three Ways

Makes: 4

Prep Time: 25 minutes

Cook Time: 10 minutes

4 large pasture-raised organic eggs per Snack Pot recipe (one egg per jar)

Eggs are one of the easiest, most nutrient-dense sources of protein. They are filled with omega-3 fats, iron, vitamins A and D, folate, and choline—to name just a few of the essential vitamins and minerals integral to our health. I love these hard-boiled egg pots because they are flavorful, quick snacks that are perfect when you're in a hurry or need a bite between meals. Here are three of my favorite flavor combinations, each providing a nutritious snack that is high in protein and flavor. Each combination yields enough for four small glass jars, fitted with lids.

Bring a pot of water to a boil over high heat. Gently add the eggs and cook for 10 minutes. With a slotted spoon, transfer the eggs to a bowl of ice water. Once cold, peel the shells and cut the eggs in half.

AVOCADO, CHILI, AND LIME

1 ripe avocado, halved, pitted, and peeled

1 tablespoon lime juice

Pinch of red pepper flakes

1 tablespoon finely chopped fresh cilantro leaves

¼ teaspoon kosher salt

Pickled Red Onions (page 210), optional

1. Mash the avocado in a bowl using a fork. Add the lime juice and pepper flakes and mash until almost smooth. Stir in the cilantro and season with salt. Divide the mixture among jars with lids and top each with two of the egg halves. Garnish with cilantro leaves and pickled onions, if desired, and close the lids tightly.

2. Store in the refrigerator for up to 2 days.

HUMMUS AND ALMOND DUKKAH

½ cup hummus (page 115, or store-bought hummus)

2 teaspoons Almond Dukkah (page 209)

1. Divide the hummus among four jars with lids. Top each with two of the egg halves. Garnish with ½ teaspoon dukkah and close the lids tightly.

2. Store in the refrigerator for up to 2 days.

SPICY HARISSA AND YOGURT

½ cup sheep's milk yogurt

1 tablespoon lemon juice

2 teaspoons harissa paste

¼ teaspoon kosher salt

⅓ cup cherry tomatoes, halved

Fresh cilantro leaves, for garnish
(optional)

1. In a small bowl, combine the
yogurt, lemon juice, harissa, and
salt and stir until well combined.
Divide the yogurt among four
jars with lids. Add some cherry
tomatoes and two egg halves to
each. Garnish with cilantro leaves,
if desired, and close the lids tightly.

2. Store in the refrigerator for
up to 2 days.

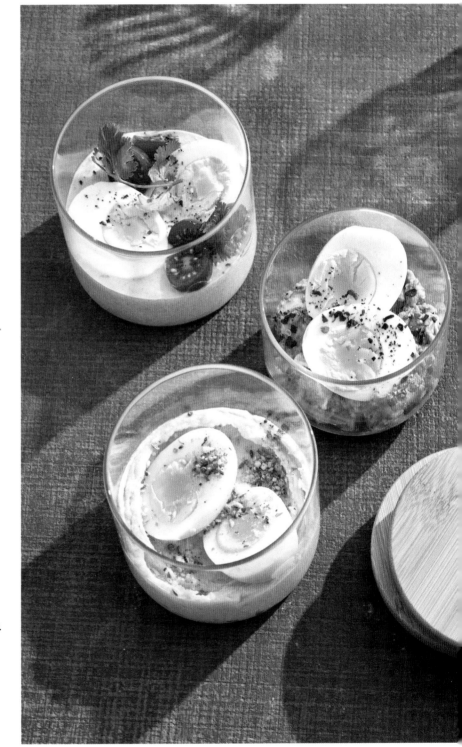

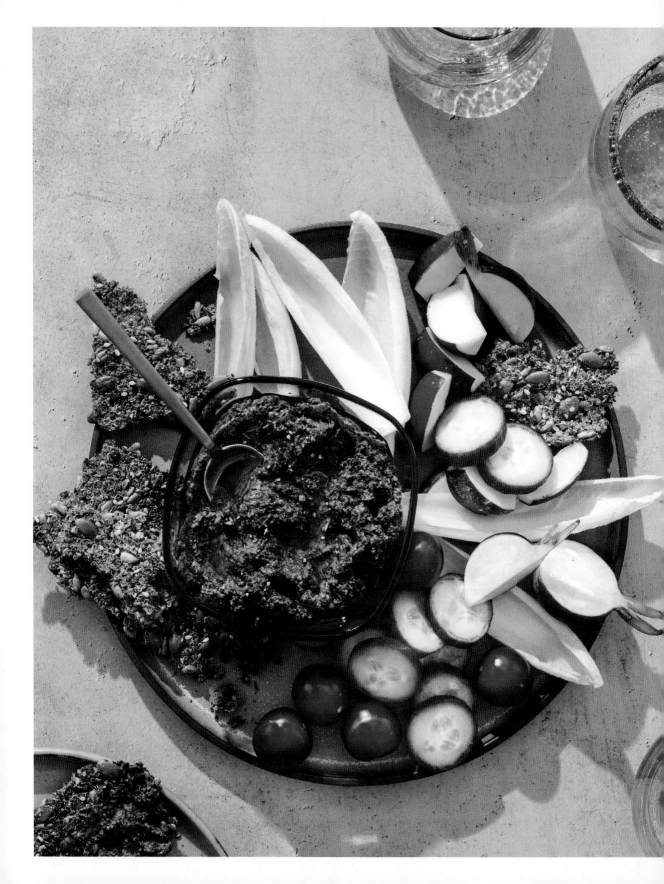

Mushroom Tapenade

Serves: 4 to 6

Prep Time: 15 minutes

Cook Time: 10 minutes

1 (½-ounce) package dried porcini mushrooms

Boiling water

1 pound cremini mushrooms, roughly chopped

1 garlic clove, minced

1 teaspoon fresh thyme leaves, plus more for garnish

1 cup pitted kalamata olives

2 tablespoons extra-virgin olive oil

1 to 2 teaspoons lemon juice, to taste

Mushrooms, one of nature's finest offerings, are rich in umami, texture, and nutrition. I use dried porcini mushrooms to boost the rich mushroom flavor of creminis, then combine them with black olives to create a delicious tapenade. Olives are rich in polyphenols and other anti-aging phytonutrients that help protect your skin, boost memory, and lower cholesterol. This is a quick and easy spread that you will want to slather over everything.

1. Place the porcini mushrooms in a heatproof bowl and cover with just boiled water. Let soak for 10 minutes, until rehydrated. Drain and rinse the porcini under clean water, roughly chop, and set aside.

2. Heat a nonstick pan over medium heat. Add the cremini mushrooms to the dry pan and cook for 5 minutes, stirring often, until they release their liquid. Add the chopped porcini along with the garlic and thyme and cook for 2 minutes, until fragrant. Remove from the heat and allow to cool slightly.

3. Transfer the mixture to a food processor, add the olives, and pulse until roughly chopped. Add 1 tablespoon of the olive oil and 1 teaspoon lemon juice and pulse until the mixture is chopped up but not smooth. Season with more lemon juice, if needed.

4. Scrape the mixture into a bowl and garnish with the remaining 1 tablespoon olive oil and additional thyme leaves.

5. Store in an airtight container in the refrigerator for up to 1 week.

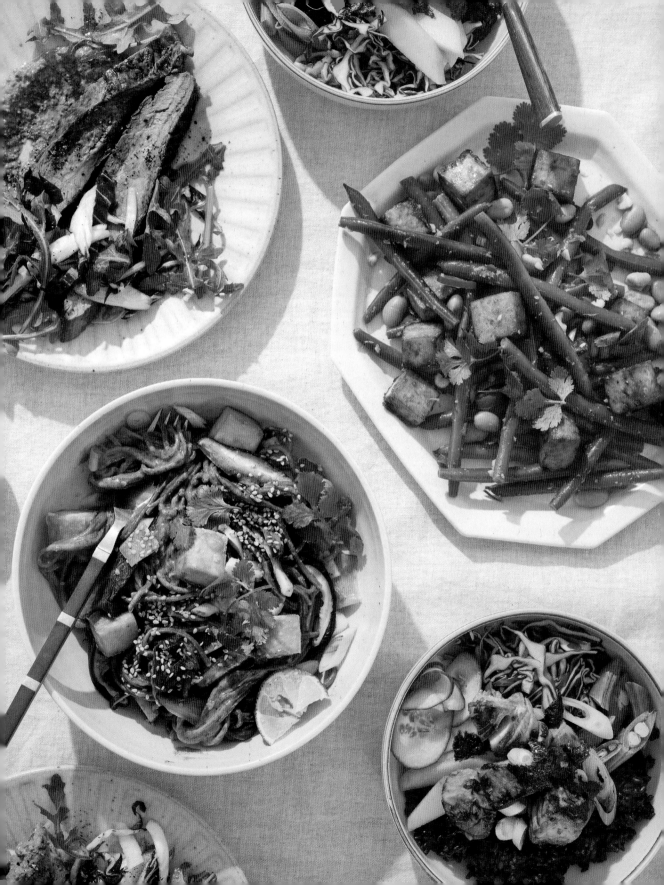

Salads and Bowls

If you're like me, you're likely always on the hunt for food that satisfies easily without feeling heavy. Something that nourishes both the body and the soul and packs in highly digestible ingredients with loads of flavor and excitement. These salads and bowls contain healthy fats, lean proteins, vitamins, and minerals, all of which actively contribute to longevity by fueling the body with essential antioxidant and anti-inflammatory effects. Some can be made in a pinch, like my Summer Tomato Salad with Smoked Mackerel (page 61); a few can be prepared ahead of time, like the Buckwheat Bowl with Smoked Paprika Chicken (page 65); and a couple may require a bit more patience but can easily feed a crowd, like my Cold Soba Noodle Salad with Mushrooms, Bok Choy, and Tofu (page 73). The variety in ingredients and flavors will take you through the seasons, and some may even earn a spot in your regular cooking repertoire.

Quinoa, Strawberry, and Sunchoke Salad

Serves: 4

Prep Time: 20 minutes

Cook Time: 45 minutes

Sunchokes

8 small sunchokes, sliced about ⅛ inch thick (about 2½ cups)

2 tablespoons extra-virgin olive oil

1 teaspoon kosher salt

½ teaspoon freshly ground black pepper

Salad

½ cup quinoa

1 cup water

1 cup quartered strawberries

⅓ cup fresh or thawed frozen peas

1 bunch kale, deveined and sliced

4 ounces sheep's milk feta cheese

¼ cup toasted pumpkin seeds

Dressing

3 tablespoons extra-virgin olive oil

1 tablespoon lemon juice

1 tablespoon apple cider vinegar

1 tablespoon grainy Dijon mustard

1 teaspoon maple syrup

½ teaspoon kosher salt

¼ teaspoon freshly ground black pepper

Sunchokes, often called Jerusalem artichokes, are nutritious tubers that are delicious when roasted. Cooking sunchokes well is important because they contain a gut-healthy prebiotic called inulin, which, although good for your digestive tract, can lead to gas and bloating if not prepared properly. Roasted sunchoke "chips" are the perfect way to avoid this, and they are absolutely delicious. Paired with sweet summer strawberries, quinoa, and peas, this wholesome salad keeps well for a few days.

1. **For the sunchokes:** Preheat the oven to 425°F. Line a baking sheet with parchment paper. Toss the sunchokes with the olive oil, salt, and pepper. Transfer to the baking sheet and roast for 25 minutes, flipping halfway through, until golden brown and crisp and the edges begin to curl. Set aside to cool.

2. Meanwhile, cook the quinoa for the salad: Bring the quinoa and water to a boil in a saucepan over medium heat. Reduce to a simmer, cover, and cook for 12 minutes, until the liquid is absorbed. Remove from the heat, fluff with a fork, and allow to cool completely.

3. **For the dressing:** In a small bowl whisk all the ingredients together.

4. **For the salad:** Toss the prepared quinoa, roasted sunchokes, strawberries, and peas together with the salad dressing. Add the kale, tossing to coat. Transfer to a platter and scatter the feta and toasted pumpkin seeds on top. Serve immediately.

Serves: 4

Prep Time: 25 minutes

Cook Time: 40 minutes

Coconut Bacon Bits

1 tablespoon coconut aminos

2 teaspoons maple syrup

1 teaspoon smoked paprika

1 cup unsweetened coconut flakes

Sweet Potato

1 medium sweet potato, peeled and cut into 1-inch cubes

2 tablespoons extra-virgin olive oil

½ teaspoon kosher salt

Dressing

1 cup loosely packed fresh cilantro leaves

2 tablespoons lime juice

2 tablespoons extra-virgin olive oil

1 tablespoon white wine vinegar

1 garlic clove, peeled

½ to 1 jalapeño pepper, seeded

1 teaspoon ground cumin

¼ teaspoon kosher salt

1 to 2 tablespoons water

Salad

4 large pasture-raised organic eggs

4 cups chopped romaine lettuce

½ cup frozen edamame, thawed

1 cup cherry tomatoes, halved

½ cup Pickled Red Onions (page 210)

8 ounces soft goat cheese, chilled and crumbled

Coconut Cobb Salad

This substantial salad, a healthful twist on the classic Cobb, is packed with nutritiously dense vegetables, protein, and a crunchy savory topping: It is bound to keep you full all day. The homemade coconut bacon bits are my favorite plant-based part of the salad. Coconut contains fiber and healthy fats and, when seasoned and toasted, it becomes a highly addictive snack or savory topping!

1. **For the coconut bacon:** Preheat the oven to 325°F. Line a baking sheet with parchment paper. In a large bowl, stir together the coconut aminos, maple syrup, and paprika. Add the coconut flakes and gently toss to combine. Spread on the baking sheet and bake, stirring every 5 minutes, for 15 minutes, until golden brown. Allow to cool completely. The bacon bits can be made ahead and stored in an airtight container for up to 5 days.

2. **For the sweet potato:** Increase the oven to 400°F. Line a baking sheet with parchment paper. In a large bowl, combine the sweet potato with the olive oil and salt. Transfer to the sheet and roast for 20 to 25 minutes, until soft and golden.

3. **For the dressing:** Combine all the ingredients in a blender and blitz until smooth, adding more water if necessary.

4. **For the eggs:** Bring a pot of water to a boil. Gently add the eggs and cook for 8 minutes. Remove and place in ice water. When cool, peel and halve the eggs.

5. **To assemble the salad:** Fill four bowls with the romaine lettuce. Divide the edamame, tomatoes, pickled onions, and sweet potato among the bowls. Top each with two hard-boiled egg halves and sprinkle some coconut bacon and crumbled goat cheese. Drizzle with the dressing and serve.

Zucchini Ribbons with Grilled Chicken and Preserved Lemon

Serves: 4

Prep Time: 20 minutes

Cook Time: 15 minutes

Dressing

2 tablespoons extra-virgin olive oil

2 tablespoons lemon juice

2 tablespoons preserved lemon, seeded, skin and flesh finely chopped

1 tablespoon tahini

1 garlic clove, grated

1 teaspoon honey

½ teaspoon kosher salt

Pinch of freshly ground black pepper

Chicken

1 pound boneless skinless pasture-raised chicken breasts

1 garlic clove, roughly chopped

2 tablespoons lemon juice

2 tablespoons extra-virgin olive oil

½ teaspoon kosher salt

½ teaspoon freshly ground black pepper

Salad

2 small zucchini, peeled into ribbons

½ pound asparagus, woody ends trimmed and stalks peeled into ribbons

½ cup pomegranate seeds

¼ cup chopped fresh mint leaves

¼ cup roughly chopped toasted pistachios

Beautiful summer zucchini is a delicious low-carb squash that can be prepared in many ways, including simply peeled into ribbons and served raw. Zucchini is packed with nutrients like vitamin C and magnesium and also contains carotenoids, which are proven to help reduce your risk for cardiovascular disease. I've paired zucchini and asparagus ribbons with tender lemony chicken for a protein and flavor boost.

The keys to this salad are to look for small zucchini, as they contain fewer seeds and water; gently use a vegetable peeler to create long ribbons of the vegetables; and wait to dress the salad until just before you're ready to serve.

1. **For the dressing:** In a small bowl, whisk all the ingredients together until smooth. Set aside.

2. **For the chicken:** Preheat the grill to 450°F or heat a grill pan over medium-high heat. Using a sharp knife, slice the chicken breasts in half horizontally, starting with the more bulbous end. Place the chicken in a nonreactive bowl and add the garlic, lemon juice, olive oil, salt, and pepper. Set aside while you prepare the salad.

3. **For the salad:** Place the zucchini and asparagus peels in a paper towel–lined bowl; this helps draw out any excess moisture. On a large platter, arrange the zucchini ribbons and asparagus curls. Sprinkle with the pomegranate seeds, mint leaves, and pistachios.

4. Grill the chicken for 5 to 7 minutes per side, until cooked through with an internal temperature of 165°F. Set aside to cool slightly, then thinly slice.

5. **To serve:** Drizzle the salad with the dressing and serve with the lemony grilled chicken.

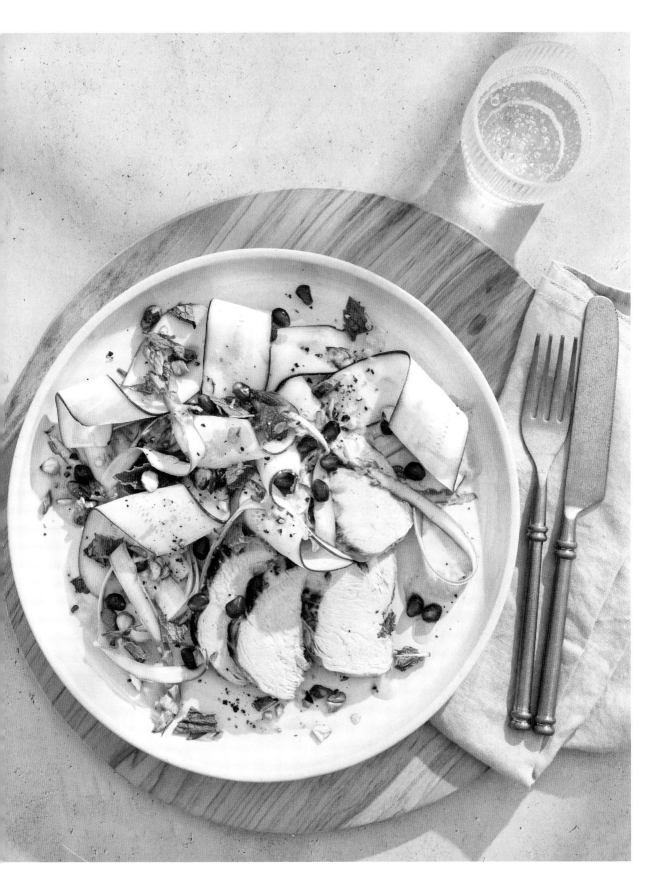

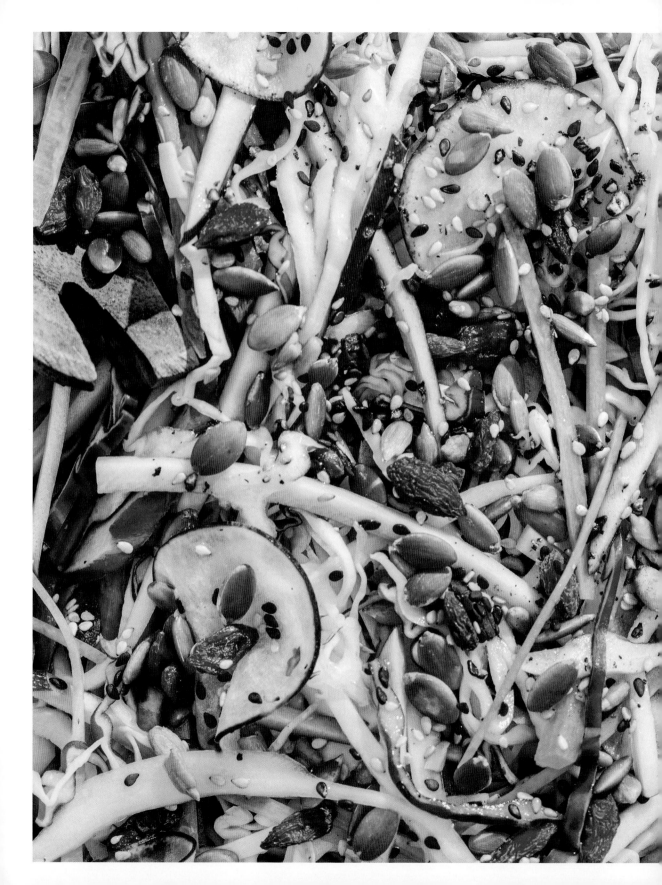

Cabbage Slaw with Savory Seed Mix

Serves: 4 to 6

Prep Time: 20 minutes

Seed Mix

½ cup goji berries

½ cup raw pumpkin seeds

¼ cup raw sunflower seeds

3 tablespoons black sesame seeds

3 tablespoons white sesame seeds

Lemon-Lime Dressing

¼ cup extra-virgin olive oil

¼ cup lime juice

2 tablespoons lemon juice

1 teaspoon honey

1 teaspoon kosher salt

½ teaspoon freshly ground black pepper

Salad

3 cups shredded white or purple cabbage

1 zucchini, julienned

1 large carrot, peeled and julienned

6 radishes, thinly sliced

This vibrant slaw, a terrific side for your summer BBQ, is a great make-ahead dish. All the components can be prepared ahead and assembled last minute. I make my seed mix in larger batches so that I have it on hand to sprinkle over salads or grilled vegetables. (Store any leftover seed mix in an airtight container in the fridge for up to 1 month.)

1. **For the seed mix:** Combine all the ingredients in a container fitted with a lid.

2. **For the dressing:** In a small bowl or large measuring cup, whisk all the ingredients together until smooth and well combined.

3. **To assemble the salad:** Mix all the salad ingredients together in a large bowl. Add enough dressing to coat. Season to taste, then sprinkle with ½ cup of the seed mix. Serve immediately.

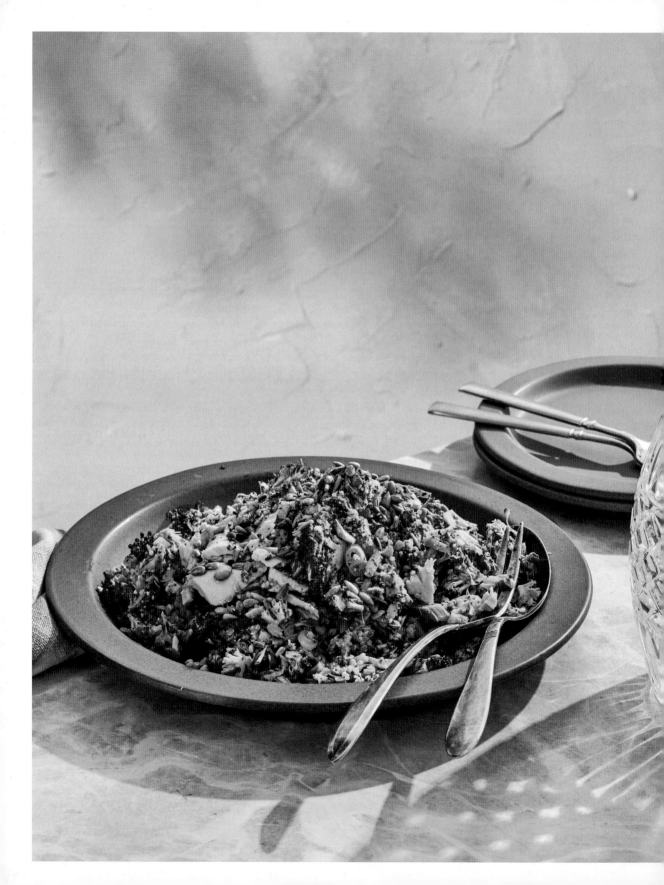

Broccoli and Quinoa Slaw with Wild Salmon and Hemp Pesto

Serves: 4 to 6

Prep Time: 15 minutes

Cook Time: 15 minutes

1 cup water

½ cup white quinoa

2 small broccoli heads, florets chopped and stems grated

1 large carrot, peeled and grated

⅓ cup thinly sliced (on the bias) scallions

⅓ cup toasted sunflower seeds

2 (5-ounce) cans sustainable wild-caught salmon

Cilantro Hemp Pesto

2 cups packed fresh cilantro leaves with soft stems

1 cup packed fresh mint leaves

½ cup hemp hearts

¼ cup lemon juice

1 garlic clove, peeled

1 teaspoon kosher salt, plus more to taste

⅓ cup extra-virgin olive oil, plus more for serving

Broccoli is one of the most delicious cruciferous vegetables out there. Packed with cancer-fighting and anti-aging compounds, fiber, and vitamins C and K, this simple vegetable can help build a strong immune system and keep your memory sharp. My favorite trick with broccoli, raw or cooked, is to use the stem! While most people discard this overlooked part, it is surprisingly tender and flavorful. Simply use a vegetable peeler to remove a few outer layers until you reach the tender core, grate or chop it up, and add it to your next stir-fry or salad. Topped with omega-rich canned wild salmon, this is a great meal you can enjoy either for lunch or dinner.

1. Bring the water and quinoa to a boil in a pot over high heat. Reduce the heat, cover, and cook for 12 minutes, until all the liquid is absorbed. Remove from the heat, fluff with a fork, and cool completely.

2. In a large mixing bowl, combine the cooked quinoa, broccoli, carrot, scallions, and half the sunflower seeds. Mix well and set aside while you make the pesto.

3. **For the pesto:** In a food processor combine the cilantro, mint, hemp hearts, lemon juice, garlic, and salt. Pulse until it forms a paste. Gradually add the olive oil until it loosens, adding a splash of water if needed.

4. Add the pesto to the slaw and mix well to combine. Divide the salad between bowls and top with salmon, the remaining sunflower seeds, a drizzle of olive oil, and salt to taste.

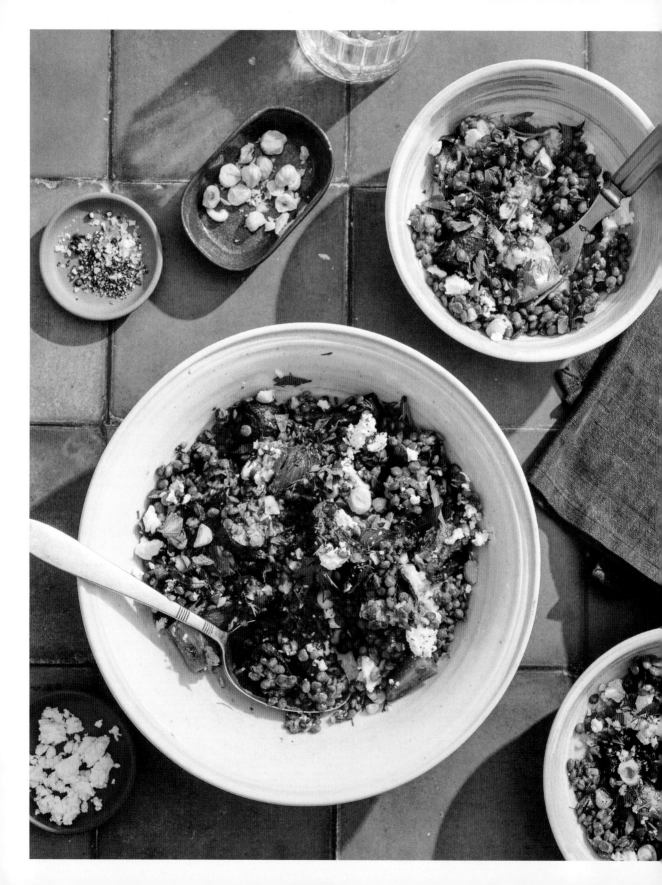

Roasted Beets with Lentils and Hazelnuts

Serves: 4 to 6

Prep Time: 20 minutes

Cook Time: 45 minutes

Hazelnut Vinaigrette

¼ cup hazelnut oil

2 tablespoons extra-virgin olive oil

3 tablespoons white wine vinegar

1 tablespoon Dijon mustard

1 small shallot, finely chopped

½ teaspoon kosher salt

¼ teaspoon freshly ground black pepper

Beets

3 large or 6 small purple, yellow, or orange beets, peeled and cut into wedges

1 large red onion, quartered

2 tablespoons avocado oil

½ teaspoon kosher salt

½ teaspoon freshly ground black pepper

Salad

¾ cup dry French green lentils (see Tip)

4 ounces sheep's or goat milk feta cheese

½ cup roughly chopped toasted hazelnuts

¼ cup chopped fresh flat-leaf parsley leaves

¼ cup chopped fresh dill

Roasting beets is a great way to maximize their flavor with minimal effort. Naturally sweet, beets become caramelized when roasted, transforming the otherwise humble veggie into something truly delicious. Beets come in a variety of colors—yellow, orange, pink, and the more common purple— all of which share the same powerful antioxidant properties.

This hearty salad, packed with protein and fiber from the lentils and folate from the beets, is great as a meal on its own or served up with grilled chicken or fish. If you can't find hazelnut oil, swap in walnut oil and toasted walnuts for an equally delicious pairing.

1. **For the hazelnut vinaigrette:** In a small bowl, whisk all of the ingredients until smooth. Set aside.

2. **For the beets:** Preheat the oven to 400°F and line a baking sheet with parchment paper. Place the beets and red onion on the baking sheet. Drizzle with avocado oil, season with salt and pepper, and toss. Roast for 45 minutes, until the beets are fork tender. Set aside to cool slightly.

3. **For the lentils:** Rinse in a fine mesh sieve and pick out any discolored ones. Place in a medium pot and cover with 2 cups water. Bring to a boil, then reduce the heat to low and simmer until they are cooked but still hold their shape, 10 to 12 minutes. Drain well.

4. **To assemble the salad:** Transfer the cooked lentils to a large bowl, add the beets and onion, and stir gently. Add the vinaigrette and mix to combine. Sprinkle with the feta cheese, hazelnuts, and fresh herbs. Serve immediately.

Tip: *French green or Puy lentils are a variety of lentils with an earthy aroma and delicious taste. They hold their shape quite well compared to other lentil varieties, which is why they are commonly used in salads and soups. If you can't find Puy lentils, a can of green lentils is a good substitute (no need to cook).*

Lentil and Spinach Salad
with Spiced Chicken

Serves: 4 to 6

Prep Time: 15 minutes

Cook Time: 20 minutes

Chicken

1½ pounds boneless skinless pasture-raised chicken breasts

1 teaspoon ground cumin

½ teaspoon kosher salt

¼ teaspoon freshly ground black pepper

1 tablespoon avocado oil

Dressing

¼ cup extra-virgin olive oil

2 tablespoons red wine vinegar

1 tablespoon Dijon mustard

1 teaspoon grated lemon zest

1 tablespoon lemon juice

1 teaspoon ground sumac, plus extra for garnish

½ teaspoon kosher salt

¼ teaspoon freshly ground black pepper

Salad

1 (15.5-ounce) can green or brown lentils, drained and rinsed

¼ English cucumber, thinly sliced

½ cup thinly sliced red onion

4 cups baby spinach

½ cup roughly chopped toasted almonds

Cumin-spiced chicken and a citrusy sumac dressing make this filling salad an excellent choice for lunch or dinner. Lentils contain essential collagen-boosting vitamins, complex carbohydrates, fiber, and protein perfect for healthy aging skin. Quickly seasoned chicken breasts are flash seared then baked, adding an extra boost of protein to this substantial salad.

1. Preheat the oven to 350°F.

2. **For the chicken:** Season the chicken with the cumin, salt, and pepper. Heat the avocado oil in a heavy cast-iron pan over medium-high heat. Add the chicken and cook for 3 to 4 minutes per side, until seared and golden. Transfer the pan to the oven and bake the chicken for 12 to 15 minutes, until it is cooked through and has an internal temperature of 165°F.

3. **For the dressing:** In a small bowl, whisk all the ingredients together.

4. **To assemble the salad:** In a large bowl, mix the lentils with the cucumber and red onion. Add a couple tablespoons of the dressing and toss to coat. Add the spinach and gently toss. Drizzle the remaining dressing over the salad and sprinkle with the toasted almonds and additional sumac, if desired.

5. Slice the chicken and serve on top of the dressed salad.

Tip: *Sumac is a citrusy, sweet, and floral spice most commonly used in Middle Eastern cooking. It can be found in most Middle Eastern grocers and gourmet food shops.*

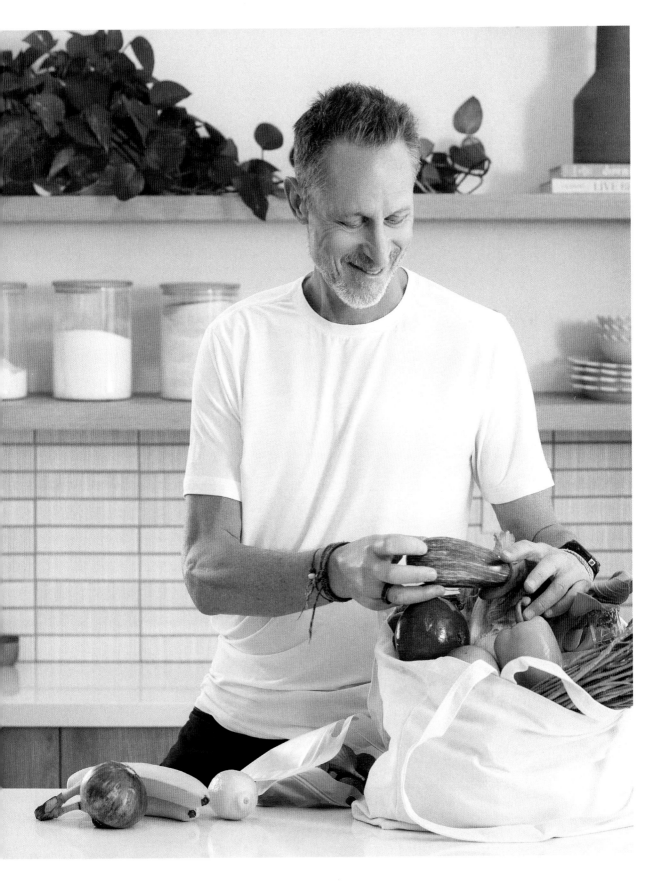

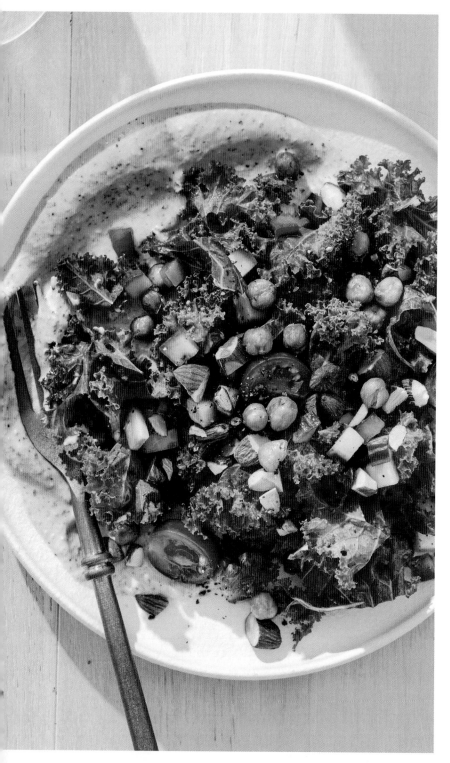

Serves: 4 to 6
Prep Time: 20 minutes
Cook Time: 25 minutes

Chickpeas

1 (15.5-ounce) can chickpeas, drained, rinsed, and well dried

2 tablespoons extra-virgin olive oil

1 teaspoon kosher salt

½ teaspoon freshly ground black pepper

Whipped Feta

8 ounces goat or sheep's milk feta cheese

1 tablespoon lime juice

½ cup loosely packed fresh mint leaves

½ cup loosely packed fresh cilantro leaves

½ to 1 jalapeño, seeded and roughly chopped

1 garlic clove, peeled

2 tablespoons sheep's milk yogurt, if needed

Chickpea Chop Salad with Whipped Jalapeño Feta

Dressing

2 tablespoons extra-virgin olive oil

2 tablespoons red wine vinegar

1 tablespoon lime juice

2 teaspoons honey

½ teaspoon kosher salt

¼ teaspoon freshly ground black pepper

Salad

1 bunch curly green kale, deveined and sliced

½ English cucumber, finely diced

1 red bell pepper, stemmed, seeded, and finely diced

1 cup halved cherry tomatoes

½ cup roughly chopped toasted almonds

Crispy baked chickpeas are a fan favorite in my household. A healthy snack on its own or tossed into a salad, they are deliciously crunchy and nutritious, with high amounts of fiber, folate, and essential B vitamins for cell health and function. I've paired them with a creamy, spicy whipped feta and crunchy green salad to make this the perfect midday meal.

1. **For the chickpeas:** Preheat the oven to 400°F. Line a baking sheet with parchment paper. In a large bowl, combine the chickpeas, olive oil, salt, and pepper. Toss to coat, then transfer to the baking sheet. Roast for 20 to 25 minutes, until golden and crisp.

2. **For the whipped feta:** In a food processor, combine the feta, lime juice, mint, cilantro, jalapeño, and garlic. Blend until smooth and whipped, about 2 minutes; stir in yogurt if the mixture is too thick.

3. **For the dressing:** In a large bowl, whisk all the ingredients together.

4. **For the salad:** Add the kale to the bowl with the dressing. Using clean hands, massage the dressing into the kale. Add the cucumber, red pepper, and tomatoes, mixing to combine. Stir in most of the chickpeas, reserving some for garnish.

5. **To serve:** Spread a heaping spoonful of the whipped feta along one side of a bowl. Add a large scoop of the salad into the center of the bowl and garnish with toasted almonds and the remaining chickpeas.

Bitter Greens with Steak and Romesco Sauce

Serves: 4

Prep Time: 20 minutes

Cook Time: 15 minutes

Steak

1¼ pounds flank or hanger steak

½ teaspoon kosher salt

¼ teaspoon freshly ground black pepper

1 tablespoon avocado oil

Romesco Sauce

1 cup roasted red peppers from a jar, drained

½ cup toasted walnuts

¼ cup fresh flat-leaf parsley leaves

1 garlic clove, peeled

1 tablespoon sherry vinegar

1 tablespoon tomato paste

1 teaspoon smoked paprika

1 teaspoon kosher salt

Pinch of red pepper flakes

2 tablespoons extra-virgin olive oil

Salad

1 small head radicchio, outer leaves removed, shredded

1 endive, outer leaves removed, sliced

2 cups baby arugula

2 tablespoons fresh lemon juice

3 tablespoons extra-virgin olive oil

Flaky sea salt and freshly ground black pepper, to taste

Juicy grilled steak topping sharp bitter greens with a smoky romesco sauce make for an absolutely stellar salad. I've swapped out the usual almonds for omega-3-rich walnuts in this Catalonian romesco made with vitamin C–rich red peppers. I like to use a hanger or flank steak, as the cooking time is quick, but you can easily use another butcher's cut such as top sirloin or strip loin.

1. **For the steak:** Preheat the oven to 350°F. Season the steak with the salt and pepper. Heat the avocado oil in a cast-iron pan over medium-high heat. Add the steak and cook, without moving it, for 3 to 4 minutes, until deeply golden on the bottom. Flip the steak and cook on the other side for 3 to 4 minutes, until deeply golden on the other side. Place the pan in the oven and roast for 5 to 7 minutes (depending on the thickness of the steak), until medium-rare, with an internal temperature of 130°F. Let rest for at least 10 minutes.

2. **For the romesco:** In a food processor, combine all the ingredients except the olive oil. Blend until smooth, scraping down the sides. With the processor running, gradually add the olive oil until smooth. Add a splash of water if the sauce is too thick.

3. **For the salad:** Mix the radicchio, endive, and arugula together in a large bowl with the lemon juice and olive oil. Season with a pinch of flaky sea salt and freshly ground black pepper.

4. Slice the steak and serve over the dressed greens with a good dollop of romesco.

Tip: *If you can, take your steak out of the fridge at least 15 minutes before you cook it. By bringing meat to room temperature, you're helping retain moisture and allowing for an even cook all the way through.*

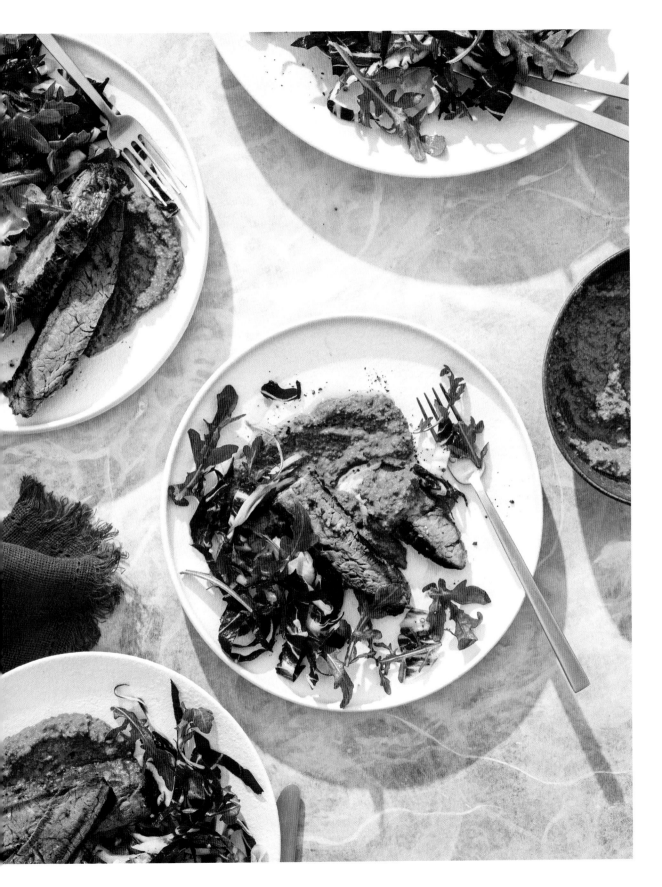

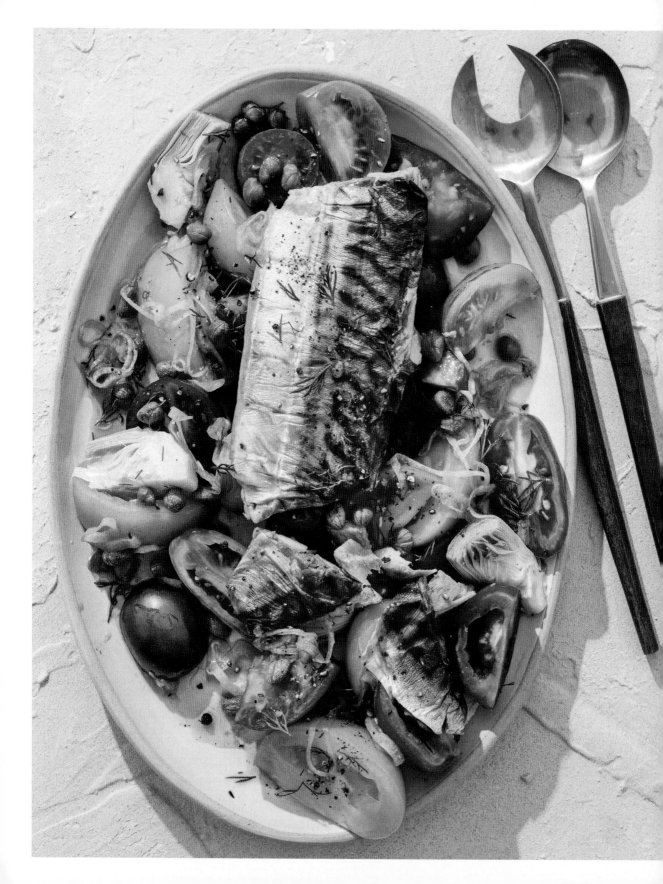

Summer Tomato Salad with Smoked Mackerel

Serves: 4

Prep Time: 10 minutes

1 shallot, thinly sliced

2 tablespoons sherry vinegar

2 tablespoons extra-virgin olive oil

½ teaspoon kosher salt

1½ pounds mixed heirloom and cherry tomatoes, cut into pieces or halved

1 (14-ounce) can artichoke hearts, drained and quartered

2 tablespoons capers, drained

¼ cup chopped fresh dill, plus more for garnish

6 ounces smoked mackerel fillet

2 tablespoons toasted pine nuts

Freshly ground black pepper, for serving

This super simple yet satisfying salad is a great example of balanced flavors. Smoky fish pairs perfectly with sweet tomatoes and bright shallots. Smoked mackerel is a flavorful ready-to-serve protein that is packed with vitamins B_{12} and D and iodine, which can help regulate thyroid hormones. Its rich flavor and high antioxidant properties can also add variety to your diet. I love to serve the salad in the late summer months when heirloom tomatoes are at their peak, but you can just use the best variety of tomatoes you can find.

1. In a small bowl, combine the shallot and sherry vinegar and let sit for 10 minutes. Whisk in the olive oil and season with salt to taste.

2. In a large bowl, toss the tomatoes with the artichokes, capers, and dill. Remove the shallots from the vinaigrette and add to the salad, tossing to coat. Top with the fillets of mackerel. Drizzle with the reserved vinaigrette and garnish with toasted pine nuts, a crack of ground black pepper, and additional dill.

Tip: *Make sure you keep your tomatoes at room temperature. This ensures the best texture because tomatoes contain an enzyme that reacts with the cold, leaving you with mushy and mealy tomatoes.*

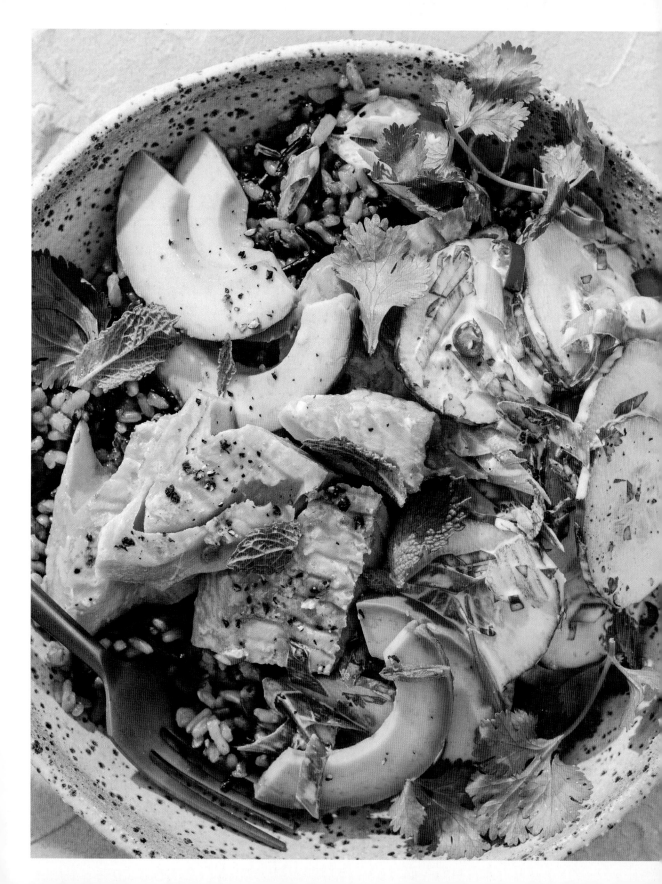

Wild Rice Bowl with Smoked Trout and Coconut Cucumber Salad

Serves: 2 to 4

Prep Time: 20 minutes

Cook Time: 45 minutes

1 cup wild rice

2 cups water

½ English cucumber, thinly sliced

4 scallions, sliced on the bias

1 small red Thai chile, seeded and finely chopped

2 tablespoons finely chopped fresh cilantro leaves, plus more for garnish

2 tablespoons finely chopped fresh mint leaves, plus more for garnish

½ cup unsweetened full-fat coconut milk

1 teaspoon grated lime zest

2 tablespoons lime juice

½ teaspoon kosher salt

5 ounces smoked trout

1 avocado, halved, pitted, and sliced

Cool, crisp cucumber often makes an appearance with smoked trout, but this time I've added a creamy coconut dressing that takes the rice bowl to the next level. Wild rice, high in protein and antioxidants, is a great base because of its chewy texture and nutty flavor, which pairs well with lightly smoked fish. Topped with sliced avocado, rich in heart-healthy monounsaturated fats that are linked with a reduced risk of cardiovascular disease, this bowl is an easy and satisfying meal. If smoked trout isn't available or you prefer another protein, the salad is great with canned salmon or grilled chicken.

1. To cook the rice, rinse it well, then place in a saucepan with the water. Bring to a boil, then reduce the heat to low and cover. Simmer until the rice is cooked but still holds its shape, 40 to 45 minutes.

2. Mix the cucumber, scallions, chile, cilantro, mint, coconut milk, lime zest and juice, and salt together until the cucumber is well coated.

3. Divide the wild rice between bowls and top with cucumber salad and pieces of smoked trout. Add a few slices of avocado and drizzle with any remaining coconut dressing. Garnish with the remaining cilantro and mint and serve.

Tip: *Cook the wild rice ahead of time to ease the prep of this dish.*

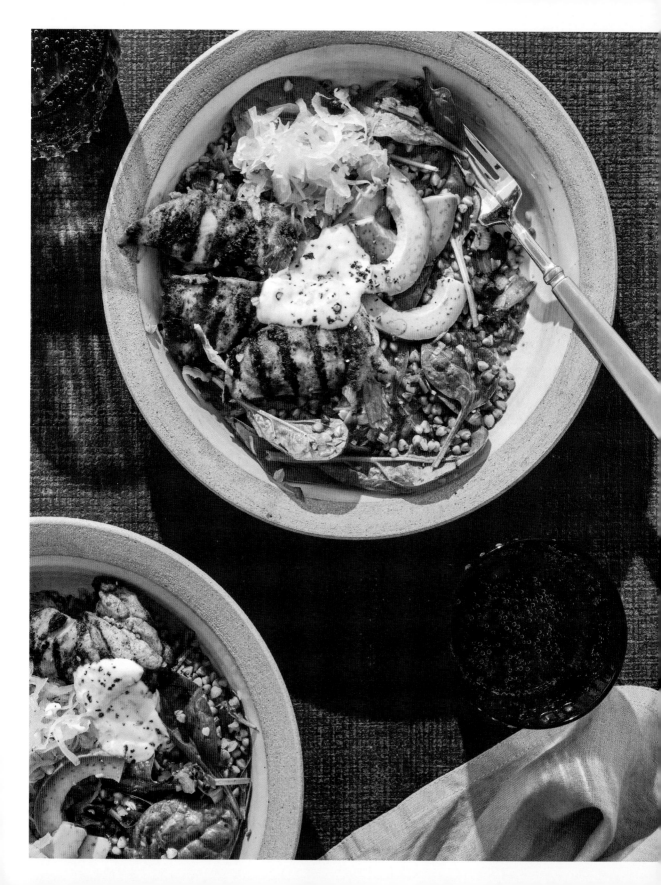

Serves: 4

Prep Time: 45 minutes,
including chilling time
Cook Time: 40 minutes

Chicken

½ cup goat or sheep's milk
yogurt, plus more for garnish

1 tablespoon extra-virgin olive oil

1 tablespoon lime juice

1 tablespoon smoked paprika

4 boneless skinless pasture-
raised chicken thighs

Salad

1 cup toasted buckwheat groats

4 cups baby spinach

1 cup sauerkraut

1 avocado, halved, pitted,
and sliced

Dressing

1 large bunch scallions, trimmed

⅓ cup extra-virgin olive oil

3 tablespoons lime juice

½ teaspoon kosher salt

1 teaspoon grated lime zest
and lime wedges, for garnish

This nutritiously dense bowl is packed with flavor and gut-friendly foods. Chicken thighs are marinated in yogurt, whose lactic acid helps tenderize the meat. The chicken is served with buckwheat groats, a unique gluten-free grain that is full of heart-healthy nutrients including magnesium, which helps the body fight off oxidative stress and chronic inflammation. Groats also contain insoluble fiber, which is particularly beneficial for gut health. Finished with fermented sauerkraut and avocado, this wholesome bowl can be prepared ahead of time and served at room temperature.

1. **To marinate the chicken:** Combine the yogurt, olive oil, lime juice, and paprika in a large nonreactive bowl. Add the chicken and coat well. Marinate in the refrigerator for at least 30 minutes, or up to 1 day.

2. **For the buckwheat groats:** Place the groats in a medium pot and cover with 2 cups water. Bring to a boil, reduce the heat to low, cover, and simmer until tender but still holding their shape, about 10 minutes. Drain excess water and set the groats aside.

3. **To grill the chicken:** Preheat the grill to 450°F (or heat a grill pan on the stove over high heat). Wipe excess marinade from the chicken and grill for 8 to 10 minutes per side, until the internal temperature reaches 165°F.

4. **For the dressing:** While the chicken is on the grill, place the scallions directly on the grill and grill for 5 to 7 minutes, until charred all over. Chop into small pieces. Transfer to a medium bowl, add the olive oil, lime juice, and salt, and mix well.

5. **For the salad:** In a large bowl, gently mix the groats and baby spinach. Add most of the charred scallion dressing, tossing to coat. Divide the groats among bowls and top with the sauerkraut, avocado, and grilled chicken. Drizzle with the remaining dressing and add a dollop of yogurt and a sprinkle of lime zest. Serve with lime wedges.

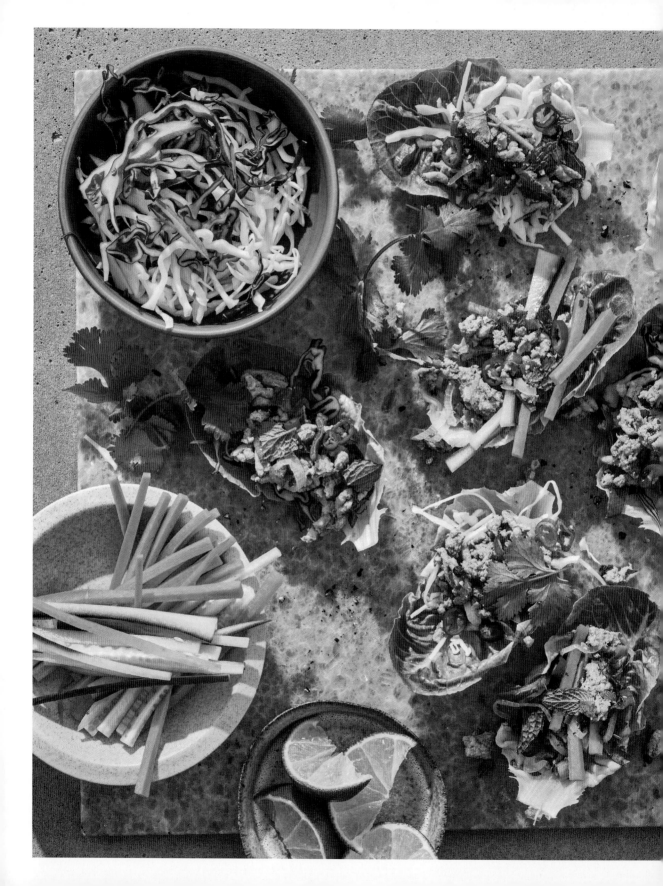

Thai Turkey Larb Lettuce Wraps

Serves: 4

Prep Time: 15 minutes
Cook Time: 15 minutes

¼ cup lime juice

2 tablespoons fish sauce

⅓ cup thinly sliced scallions

1 red Thai chile, seeded and finely chopped

¼ cup chicken stock or water

1 pound ground turkey

1 large shallot, thinly sliced

½ cup torn fresh mint leaves

½ cup fresh cilantro leaves, roughly chopped

1 to 2 Little Gem or cos lettuce heads, leaves separated

½ English cucumber, cut into thin matchsticks

1 cup shredded white or purple cabbage

1 large carrot, peeled and julienned

1 lime, cut into wedges

Larb is a traditional northern Thai dish most commonly made with pork. I've opted for a leaner protein here, but it's just as delicious! Seasoned with spicy Thai chiles, zesty lime, and bright herbs, this is a great high-protein meal that comes together quickly. I love to serve the larb in lettuce cups and let diners pick and choose their own garnishes.

1. In a large bowl, combine the lime juice, fish sauce, scallions, and chile; set the sauce aside.

2. Heat a large pan over medium heat. Add the chicken stock and ground turkey and cook for 5 minutes, using a wooden spoon to break the meat into smaller pieces as it begins to brown. Add the shallot and cook for another 4 minutes, until the shallot has softened and the turkey is no longer pink throughout. Cool for 5 minutes. Add the turkey to the sauce and toss to combine. Stir in the mint and cilantro.

3. Arrange the lettuce cups on a platter, fill with scoops of turkey larb, and add cucumber, cabbage, and carrot for garnish. Serve with lime wedges.

Tip: *Add a drizzle of peanut sauce for some extra oomph!*

Forbidden Rice and Salmon Poke Bowl

Serves: 4

Prep Time: 20 minutes

Cook Time: 35 minutes

1 cup black rice

1¾ cups water

Salmon

¼ cup gluten-free tamari or coconut aminos

2 tablespoons rice wine vinegar

2 tablespoons mirin

2 tablespoons sriracha

1 tablespoon grated fresh ginger

2 teaspoons sesame oil

1 pound sustainably caught salmon, cubed

Bowls

1 cup shredded purple cabbage

1 cup snap peas, cut into thirds

1 mango, peeled, pitted, and thinly sliced

1 tablespoon toasted sesame seeds

⅓ cup thinly sliced scallions

1 large sheet nori, torn into pieces

½ cup Quick Pickled Cucumbers (page 212)

Traditionally served with raw fish, poke bowls are a Hawaiian staple. I've switched things up by marinating cubed salmon, high in omega-3 fats, in a sweet and spicy sauce that caramelizes when the salmon is cooked. Served on a bed of black rice, which is high in antioxidants from a blackish-purple pigment called anthocyanin, then topped off with quick pickled cucumbers, sweet mango, and crunchy snap peas, it's a tasty tropical meal easy enough to whip up for lunch or dinner.

1. Rinse the black rice well, then place in a pot with the water. Bring to a boil over high heat, then reduce to a simmer, cover, and cook for 30 minutes, until tender.

2. To marinate the salmon: In a large bowl, whisk together the tamari, vinegar, mirin, sriracha, ginger, and sesame oil. Add the salmon, toss to coat, and set aside for 5 minutes.

3. Heat a large nonstick pan over medium heat. Add the cubed salmon and cook for 4 to 5 minutes, stirring frequently, until the flesh is firm and the sauce becomes slightly sticky.

4. To assemble the bowls: Add a large scoop of black rice to each bowl and top with salmon, cabbage, snap peas, and mango. Garnish with sesame seeds, scallions, nori, and a few slices of pickled cucumber.

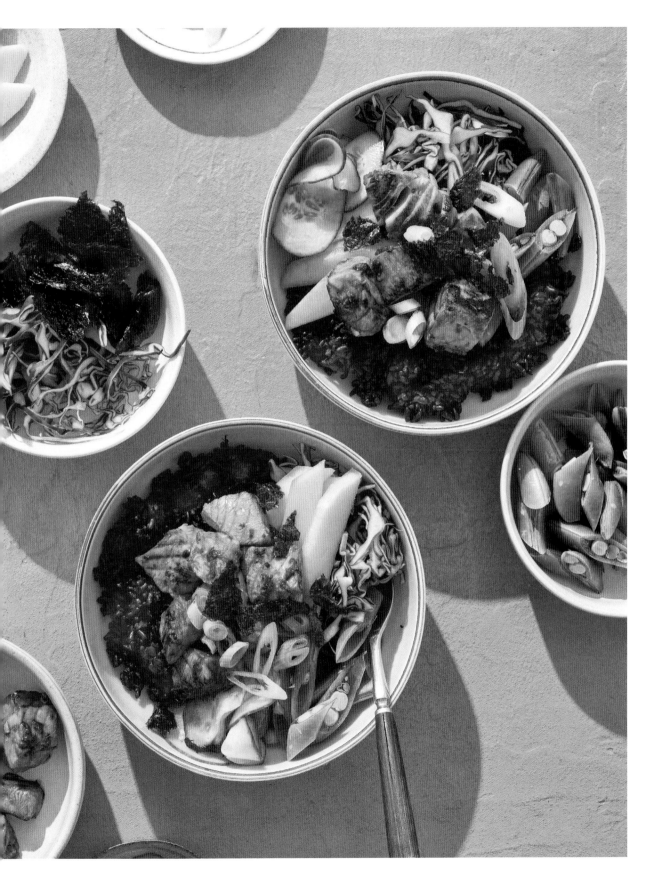

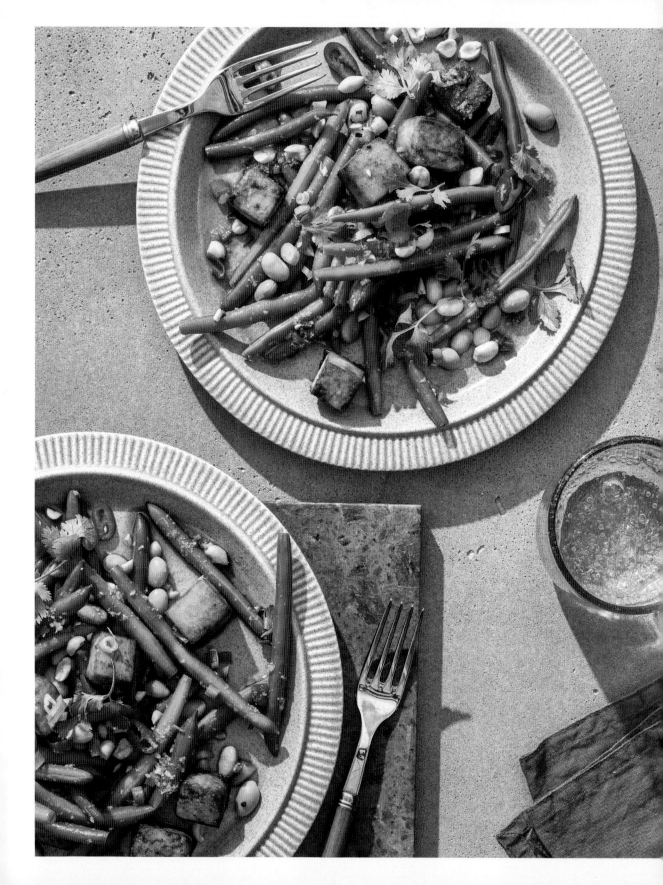

Edamame and Bean Salad with Crispy Tofu

Serves: 4

Prep Time: 30 minutes

Cook Time: 25 minutes

Tofu

1 (12-ounce) block organic extra-firm tofu, cut into 1-inch-thick slices

2 tablespoons gluten-free tamari

1 teaspoon sriracha or other hot sauce

1 tablespoon arrowroot powder or cornstarch

1 tablespoon avocado oil

Salad

1 pound green beans, trimmed

3 tablespoons rice wine vinegar

2 tablespoons lime juice

1 tablespoon avocado oil

1 tablespoon gluten-free tamari

1 teaspoon sesame oil

1 garlic clove, minced

2 teaspoons grated fresh ginger

1 cup frozen edamame, thawed

2 long red chiles, seeded; one minced, one sliced for garnish

1 bunch scallions, thinly sliced

⅓ cup roughly chopped fresh cilantro leaves

⅓ cup roughly chopped toasted peanuts or cashews

Baking tofu until crispy is one of my favorite ways to prepare the plant-based protein. Draining excess moisture from the tofu yields the crispiest cubes. I've paired these delicious morsels with a crunchy, fresh edamame and green bean salad tossed in a lime, ginger, and sesame dressing. This salad is a vegetarian powerhouse, providing ample protein and fiber and perfect for a simple meal.

1. Preheat the oven to 400°F. Line a baking sheet with parchment paper.

2. **For the tofu:** Arrange the tofu slices on a clean kitchen towel or paper towels. Cover with another kitchen towel (or paper towels) and place a heavy pan on top. Let the tofu drain for at least 15 minutes.

3. Cut the tofu into cubes. In a large bowl, whisk the tamari and sriracha until smooth. Add the tofu pieces, toss, and marinate for 10 minutes.

4. In a small bowl, whisk the arrowroot powder and avocado oil until smooth. Add to the tofu pieces, toss to coat, and arrange on the baking sheet in an even layer. Bake for 20 to 25 minutes, flipping halfway, until golden brown.

5. **For the salad:** Bring a large pot of water to a boil. Add the green beans and blanch for 3 minutes, then transfer to a bowl filled with ice water. Once cool, lift out and place on a paper towel–lined tray to drain.

6. In a large bowl, whisk together the vinegar, lime juice, avocado oil, tamari, sesame oil, garlic, and ginger. Add the blanched beans along with the edamame and toss to coat. Add the minced chile, scallions, and cilantro and mix well. Top with the crispy tofu, garnish with the toasted peanuts and sliced red chile, and serve immediately.

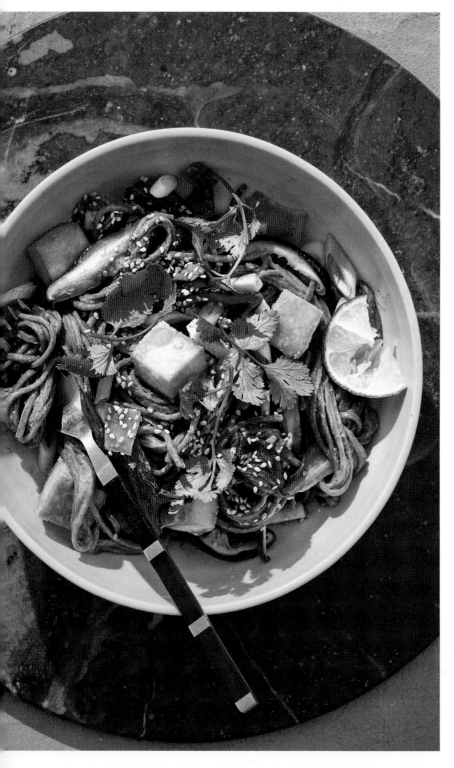

Serves: 4 to 6

Prep Time: 30 minutes

Cook Time: 35 minutes

Tofu

1 (12-ounce) block organic extra-firm tofu, cut into 1-inch-thick slices

1 tablespoon arrowroot powder

1 tablespoon avocado oil

8 ounces buckwheat soba noodles

1 teaspoon sesame oil

1 medium zucchini, halved crosswise and julienned

Mushrooms

1 teaspoon sesame oil

4½ cups sliced shiitake mushrooms

4 heads bok choy, roughly chopped

2 garlic cloves, thinly sliced

1 tablespoon gluten-free tamari

Dressing

½ cup smooth almond butter

1 tablespoon grated fresh ginger

¼ cup warm water

2 tablespoons lime juice

1 tablespoon maple syrup

1 tablespoon gluten-free tamari

1 teaspoon sesame oil

1 teaspoon sriracha

Garnish

1 cup roughly chopped fresh cilantro leaves

⅓ cup thinly sliced scallions

2 tablespoons toasted sesame seeds

This is a hearty, plant-based, gluten-free meal that is full of flavor. Mushrooms are one of the most beneficial foods out there. Shiitakes in particular are full of polysaccharide compounds that protect your immune system and provide anti-inflammatory properties. I love to serve mushrooms with crispy tofu for textural contrast, then drizzle with a creamy, nutty sauce that you'll want to pour over everything!

1. Preheat the oven to 400°F. Line a baking sheet with parchment paper.

2. **For the tofu:** Arrange the tofu slices on a clean kitchen towel or paper towels. Cover with another kitchen towel (or paper towels) and place a heavy pan on top. Let the tofu drain for at least 15 minutes.

3. Cut the tofu into cubes. In a large bowl, mix the arrowroot powder and avocado oil until no clumps remain. Add the tofu pieces and toss to coat. Transfer to the baking sheet and bake, flipping halfway through, for 20 to 25 minutes, until crispy but still tender to touch.

4. **For the noodles:** Bring a large pot of water to a boil over high heat. Add the soba noodles and cook until tender, about 6 minutes. Drain the noodles and transfer to a large bowl of ice water. Once cool, drain, transfer to a large bowl, add the sesame oil, and toss so the noodles don't stick. Add the julienned zucchini to the bowl and set aside.

5. **For the mushrooms:** Heat the sesame oil in a large nonstick pan over medium heat. Add the mushrooms and cook until they begin to soften, about 4 minutes. Add the bok choy and cook for 2 to 3 minutes. Stir in the garlic and tamari, remove from the heat, and let cool slightly. Add to the bowl of noodles and stir to combine.

6. **For the dressing:** Meanwhile, in a small bowl, whisk the almond butter and ginger with the warm water until smooth. Whisk in the lime juice, maple syrup, tamari, sesame oil, and sriracha.

7. **To serve:** Drizzle some of the dressing over the noodle mixture, tossing to coat. Top with the tofu pieces then sprinkle with the cilantro, scallions, and sesame seeds. Serve with extra dressing on the side.

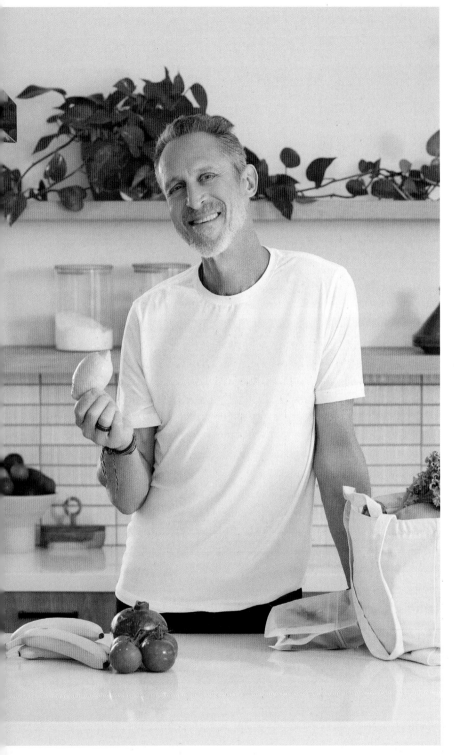

Serves: 4

Prep Time: 20 minutes

Cook Time: 25 minutes

Cauliflower Rice

1 head cauliflower, cored and roughly chopped

1 tablespoon avocado oil

2 garlic cloves, minced

½ teaspoon kosher salt

¼ cup finely chopped fresh cilantro leaves, plus more for garnish

Black-Eyed Peas

1 tablespoon avocado oil

½ cup finely chopped red onion

1 cup sliced roasted red peppers from a jar, drained

1 (15.5-ounce) can black-eyed peas, drained and rinsed

1 teaspoon ground cumin

½ teaspoon kosher salt

Cauliflower Rice Burrito Bowl

Guacamole

1 avocado, halved, pitted, and peeled

2 tablespoons lime juice

1 tablespoon finely chopped red onion

1 tablespoon finely chopped fresh cilantro

½ teaspoon kosher salt

Dressing

¼ cup extra-virgin olive oil

3 tablespoons lime juice

1 whole chipotle pepper in adobo sauce, chopped

½ teaspoon kosher salt

Pinch of freshly ground black pepper

1 lime, cut into wedges

This is my take on a burrito bowl, but healthier! Subbing in for white rice, low-carb roasted cauliflower rice is one of the most versatile kitchen hacks. It absorbs flavors well, and roasting it helps rid it of its otherwise wet texture. Heart-healthy guacamole, protein-rich black-eyed peas, and a smoky chipotle dressing complete this tasty vegan meal.

1. **For the cauliflower rice:** Preheat the oven to 425°F and line a baking sheet with parchment paper.

2. Fill a food processor about halfway with cauliflower. Pulse until it breaks down into a texture that resembles rice. Pour the contents into a large bowl and continue with the remaining cauliflower. Add the avocado oil, garlic, and salt to the cauliflower, mixing well to coat. Spread on the lined baking sheet in an even layer. Bake the cauliflower, mixing well halfway through, for 20 to 25 minutes, until golden. Stir in the cilantro and set aside.

3. **For the black-eyed peas:** Heat the avocado oil in a large pan over medium heat. Add the red onion and cook for 2 minutes, until slightly softened. Add the red peppers, black-eyed peas, cumin, and salt and mix well. Cook for about 5 minutes, until the beans are warmed through.

4. **For the guacamole:** In a bowl, mash the avocado with the lime juice, red onion, cilantro, and salt.

5. **For the dressing:** In a blender or food processor combine all the ingredients and blend until smooth.

6. **Assemble the bowls:** Divide the cauliflower rice among bowls. Top with black-eyed peas and guacamole. Drizzle with the chipotle dressing and garnish with cilantro and lime wedges.

Tip: *Freeze any extra uncooked cauliflower rice and simply defrost in a pan over medium heat.*

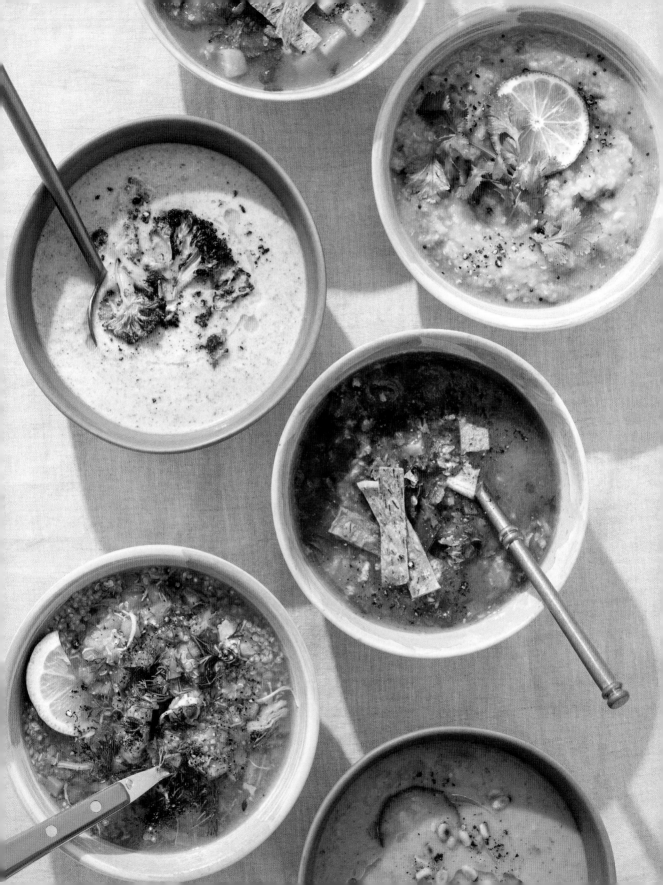

Soups and Stews

Nothing says comfort on a chilly day like a warm bowl of soup. Soups are simple and inexpensive to make, but to maximize flavor, you do need a bit of time. That means the recipes in this chapter may require some patience, but they are also a great option for batch cooking. Soups and stews are the first step to intuitive cooking, as you learn to season as you go and create the best medley of flavors. Getting a feeling for adding a little seasoning here and there can help you become a better home cook. Highly nutritious, packed with antioxidants and protein, these warming soups and stews provide tasty meals that can improve your longevity and reduce your risk for age-related disease. Whether you're looking for something substantial like Chipotle Bison Chili (page 93) or a way to use up leftover vegetables, as with Fennel Minestrone (page 79), I bet there's a soup or stew in this chapter that will absolutely win you and your family over.

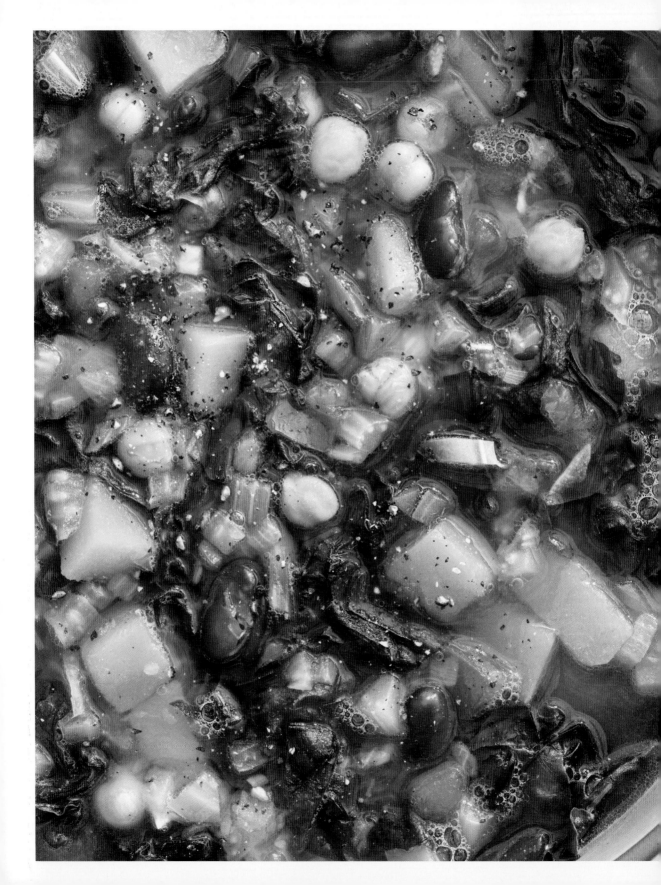

Fennel Minestrone

Serves: 4 to 6

Prep Time: 15 minutes

Cook Time: 1 hour 25 minutes

1 tablespoon extra-virgin olive oil, plus more for serving

1 yellow onion, diced

1 small fennel bulb, cored and diced

2 celery stalks, diced

½ teaspoon crushed fennel seeds

2 garlic cloves, thinly sliced

½ medium butternut squash, peeled and cubed

1 large tomato, diced

1 cup canned kidney beans, drained and rinsed

1 cup canned chickpeas, drained and rinsed

6 cups vegetable stock

1 bay leaf

2 teaspoons kosher salt

1 teaspoon freshly ground black pepper

1 small bunch Swiss chard, deveined and sliced

Grated pecorino cheese, for serving (optional)

Minestrone, or Italian-style vegetable soup, is one of the best ways to use up the odds and ends in your fridge. My addition of fennel adds a delicious hint of anise flavor. Fennel is one of the most unassuming vegetables, but it's loaded with potassium and folate and can be eaten raw, roasted, or braised. In addition to its heart-friendly nutrients, fennel contains protective polyphenols, which can help fight inflammation. I love to fill my minestrone soups with other healthful ingredients, such as protein-rich beans and vitamin A–rich Swiss chard.

1. Heat the olive oil in a large pot over medium-high heat. Add the onion, diced fennel, and celery and cook until softencd, about 5 minutes. Reduce the heat slightly, add the fennel seeds and garlic, and stir until fragrant, about 30 seconds. Add the squash and mix well. Cook over medium heat for 3 to 4 minutes.

2. Add the tomato, kidney beans, chickpeas, and stock and bring the soup to a boil. Reduce to a simmer and add the bay leaf, salt, and pepper. Simmer for 1 hour, uncovered, until the vegetables are tender. Add the Swiss chard and continue cooking for another 10 minutes, until it has softened.

3. Fish out and discard the bay leaf. Serve the soup in bowls topped with freshly grated pecorino cheese, if you like, and a drizzle of olive oil.

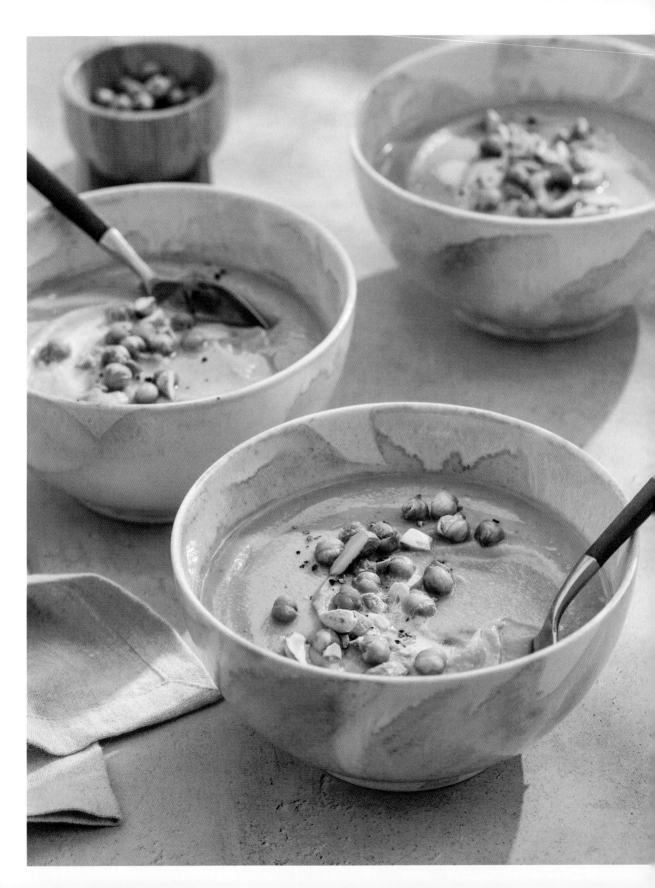

Coconut Carrot Soup with Crispy Chickpeas

Serves: 4

Prep Time: 15 minutes

Cook Time: 45 minutes

Chickpeas

1 (15.5-ounce) can chickpeas, drained, rinsed, and well dried

1 tablespoon avocado oil

2 teaspoons ground coriander

1 teaspoon kosher salt

Soup

1 tablespoon avocado oil

1 yellow onion, diced

2 pounds carrots, peeled and chopped

1 tablespoon chopped fresh ginger

2 garlic cloves, smashed

¼ cup loosely packed fresh cilantro, stems finely chopped and leaves reserved

2 teaspoons garam masala

1 teaspoon ground turmeric

½ teaspoon ground coriander

1 teaspoon kosher salt

1 (13.5-ounce) can full-fat unsweetened coconut milk, ¼ cup reserved for serving

2 to 3 cups vegetable stock or water, as needed

⅓ cup roughly chopped toasted cashews

Pureed carrot soup can seem a bit uninspiring, but this soup is packed with warm curry spices like turmeric and garam masala, along with cooling coconut to balance any heat. Turmeric is a potent spice, containing a powerful compound called curcumin, which aids in the prevention of degenerative disease. Topped with crunchy chickpeas, a healthy and protein-filled alternative to croutons, this soup is a flavorsome meal.

1. **For the chickpeas:** Preheat the oven to 400°F. Line a baking sheet with parchment paper. Toss the chickpeas in a large bowl with the avocado oil, coriander, and salt. Spread out on the baking sheet and roast for 20 to 25 minutes, until golden and crisp.

2. **For the soup:** Meanwhile, heat the avocado oil in a large pot over medium-high heat. Add the onion and cook for 3 to 4 minutes, until translucent. Add the carrots, stir, and continue cooking for another 5 minutes. Reduce the heat to low, stir in the ginger, garlic, and cilantro stems, and cook until fragrant. Stir in the garam masala, turmeric, and coriander, season with salt, and mix well.

3. Add the coconut milk and enough stock to cover. Bring to a boil, reduce to a simmer, and cover. Simmer for 30 minutes, until the carrots are fork-tender.

4. Puree the soup with an immersion blender in the pot, or in small batches in a blender, until smooth.

5. Serve topped with crispy chickpeas, cilantro leaves, a drizzle of reserved coconut milk, and a sprinkle of toasted cashews.

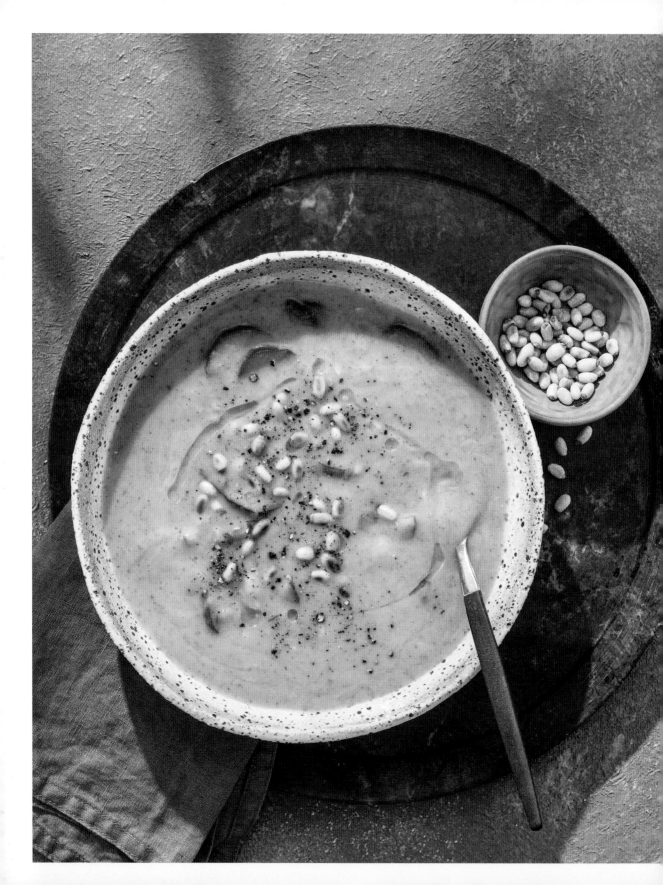

Creamy Zucchini Bean Soup

Serves: 4 to 6

Prep Time: 15 minutes

Cook Time: 50 minutes

1 (15.5-ounce) can cannellini beans, drained and rinsed

4 cups chicken or vegetable stock

2 tablespoons extra-virgin olive oil, plus more for serving

2 leeks, white and light green parts only, thinly sliced

2½ pounds (about 6 medium) zucchini, halved lengthwise and sliced

2 garlic cloves, sliced

2 teaspoons kosher salt

½ teaspoon freshly ground black pepper

½ cup fresh basil leaves, torn

1 tablespoon lemon juice

⅓ cup toasted pine nuts

The best time of year to make this soup is early in the season when zucchini is at its prime. I love to cook with zucchini because it's such a versatile, low-carbohydrate squash that can be eaten both raw and cooked, and it's packed with vitamin C and fiber, which can prevent oxidative stress caused by free radicals. This recipe is a great example of maximizing flavor by cooking zucchini until it's golden and jammy.

1. In a blender, puree the beans with 2 cups of the stock. Set aside.

2. Heat the olive oil in a large pot over medium heat. Add the leeks and cook until softened and translucent, about 4 minutes. Add the zucchini, garlic, and 1 teaspoon of the salt. Cook, stirring often, for 15 to 20 minutes, until the zucchini have turned golden and soft.

3. Add the remaining 1 teaspoon salt and the pepper, then the pureed beans and remaining 2 cups stock. Stir in the basil leaves and bring to a boil. Reduce to a simmer and cook, uncovered, for about 15 minutes.

4. Transfer two-thirds of the mixture to a food processor or blender and blend until smooth. Return the pureed soup to the pot and stir in the lemon juice. Serve with pine nuts and a good drizzle of olive oil.

Quick Spicy Tomato Soup

Serves: 4

Prep Time: 10 minutes

Cook Time: 40 minutes

2 tablespoons extra-virgin olive oil

1 yellow onion, coarsely chopped

1 large carrot, peeled and coarsely chopped

1 celery stalk, coarsely chopped

1½ teaspoons kosher salt

½ teaspoon freshly ground black pepper

2 garlic cloves, smashed

½ teaspoon red pepper flakes

1 tablespoon tomato paste

1 (28-ounce) can San Marzano or other good-quality whole tomatoes

1 (15.5-ounce) can cannellini beans, drained and rinsed

2 cups vegetable stock or water

¼ cup toasted pumpkin seeds

This speedy soup will be your new favorite staple. It's a classic tomato soup with a hint of spice as well as creaminess from beans. Cooked tomatoes contain lycopene, a carotenoid antioxidant that's known to help control cholesterol and protect against free radicals.

1. Heat the olive oil in a large pot over medium heat. Add the onion, carrot, and celery and season with the salt and pepper. Cook, stirring often, until the onion is translucent, 6 to 8 minutes.

2. Add the garlic and red pepper flakes and stir until fragrant, about a minute. Stir in the tomato paste. Add the tomatoes with their juices and cook for 5 minutes. Use a wooden spoon to break them down. Add the beans and stock, bring to a boil, then reduce the heat and simmer for 20 minutes.

3. Remove from the heat and puree with an immersion blender in the pot, or in small batches in a blender, until smooth. Top with pumpkin seeds and serve.

Curried Butternut Squash Soup

Serves: 6

Prep Time: 15 minutes

Cook Time: 30 minutes

1 tablespoon avocado oil

4 shallots, thinly sliced

2 garlic cloves, sliced

1 tablespoon chopped fresh ginger

1 (3-pound) butternut squash, peeled and roughly chopped

1 medium carrot, peeled and roughly chopped

4 to 5 cups vegetable stock or water

1 cup full-fat unsweetened coconut milk, plus more for serving

1 cup dried red lentils, rinsed well

2 tablespoons Thai red curry paste

1 teaspoon kosher salt, plus more to taste

1 to 2 teaspoons fish sauce (optional)

½ cup roughly chopped toasted cashews

Fresh cilantro leaves, for garnish

Lime wedges, for serving

This curried squash soup is a riff on one of my favorite Thai dishes, khao soi, a rich coconut curry broth typically served with egg noodles. Here I use a store-bought curry paste to punch up the flavor, and red lentils for an added nutritional boost from fiber and protein. I often treat the leftovers of this creamy, dairy-free soup as a curry, serving it with brown or wild rice for a more substantial meal.

1. Heat the avocado oil in a large pot over medium-low heat. Add the shallots, garlic, and ginger and cook, stirring, until softened, about 4 minutes. Add the squash and carrot and cook for another 5 minutes, until they begin to soften.

2. Stir in the stock, coconut milk, lentils, and curry paste. Season with salt and bring to a boil. Reduce to a simmer, cover, and cook for 15 minutes, until the vegetables and lentils are soft.

3. Remove from the heat and puree with an immersion blender in the pot, or in small batches in a blender, until smooth. Add fish sauce to taste, if using. Garnish with toasted cashews, a drizzle of reserved coconut milk, and cilantro leaves and serve with lime wedges.

Tip: *Freeze extra coconut milk in an airtight container. Simply defrost before use or add frozen to a smoothie.*

Vegan Broccoli and "Cheese" Soup

Serves 4 to 6

Prep Time: 15 minutes

Cook Time: 40 minutes

1 cup raw cashews

2¾ teaspoons kosher salt

1 cup boiling water

3 tablespoons extra-virgin olive oil

1 leek, chopped

1 yellow onion, chopped

2 garlic cloves, smashed

2 pounds broccoli, stems and crown roughly chopped, 2 cups of the chopped florets set aside

1 teaspoon freshly ground black pepper

4 cups vegetable stock or water

½ cup nutritional yeast

This vegan version of the classic broccoli soup gets its creaminess from cashew cream, while the cheesy flavor comes from nutritional yeast. I always use broccoli stalks in my cooking: Simply use a vegetable peeler to remove the tough outer layer around the stalk, then chop up the tender center. Broccoli is a delicious superfood, containing sulforaphane, the phytochemical that is responsible for the vegetable's bitter taste but also contains cancer-fighting properties.

1. Preheat the oven to 400°F. Line a baking sheet with parchment paper.

2. Place the cashews in a blender. Add ½ teaspoon of the salt and the boiling water and allow the mixture to sit for at least 5 minutes. Blend until smooth, adding ¼ to ½ cup water as needed to achieve a thickened, creamy texture similar to that of coconut milk. Set the cashew cream aside.

3. Heat 2 tablespoons of the olive oil in a large pot over medium-low heat. Add the leek, onion, and garlic and sauté until softened, 4 to 6 minutes. Season with 1 teaspoon of the salt. Add the broccoli stems and cook for 2 to 3 minutes. Add the chopped broccoli florets and continue cooking for 3 to 4 minutes. Season with 1 teaspoon of the salt and the black pepper.

4. Add the stock and stir in the nutritional yeast. Cover the pot and bring to a boil. Reduce to a simmer and cook, covered, until the broccoli is tender, 20 to 25 minutes.

5. Meanwhile, toss the reserved chopped florets with the remaining 1 tablespoon olive oil and season with the remaining ¼ teaspoon salt. Transfer to the baking sheet and roast for 20 minutes, until crisp.

6. Remove the soup from the heat and stir in ½ cup of the cashew cream. Blend with an immersion blender in the pot, or in small batches in a blender, until smooth.

7. Serve soup topped with crispy broccoli florets and a swirl of the remaining cashew cream.

Tip: *Store the extra cashew cream in an airtight container in the fridge for up to 5 days. It's delicious stirred into salad dressings or blended into smoothies for an additional protein boost.*

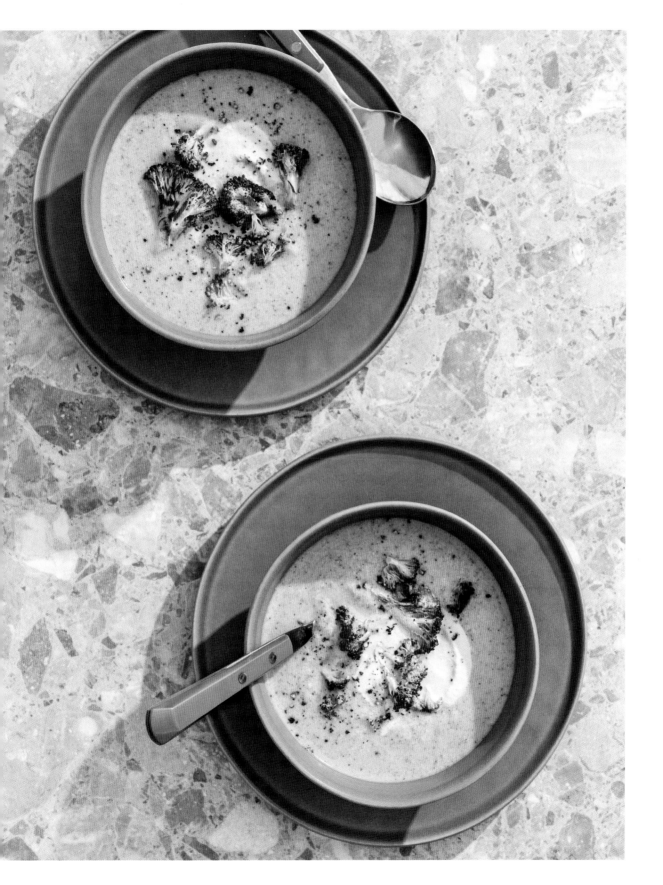

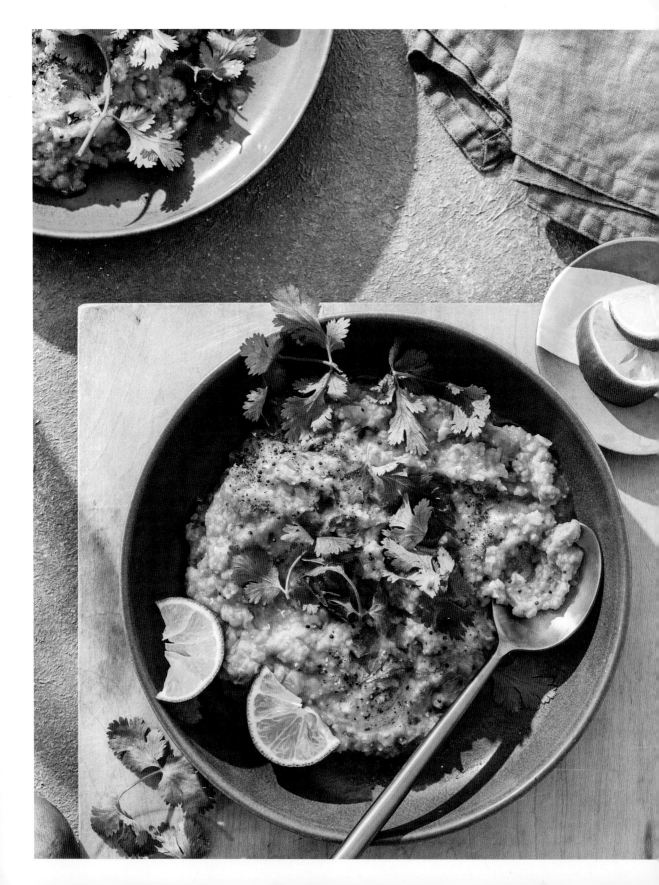

Red Lentil Tarka Dahl

Serves: 2 to 4

Prep Time: 15 minutes

Cook Time: 35 minutes

2 cups red lentils, rinsed well

4½ cups water

1 heaping teaspoon ground turmeric

1 teaspoon kosher salt

1 tablespoon avocado oil

1 teaspoon coriander seeds

1 teaspoon cumin seeds

1 teaspoon fennel seeds

1 teaspoon black mustard seeds

1 small red onion, diced

2 garlic cloves, thinly sliced

2 tablespoons finely chopped fresh ginger

1 tablespoon finely chopped fresh cilantro stems

1 large tomato, roughly chopped

1 teaspoon kosher salt

Fresh cilantro leaves, for garnish

1 lime, cut into wedges, for serving

This comforting stew is perfect for those cooler nights. Red lentil dahl is an immune-boosting, anti-aging meal on its own as it is packed with anti-inflammatory antioxidants like turmeric and fennel seed. Tarka is the technique of frying spices to unlock their aromas. Stirred into the dahl, the tarka adds nice crunch and flavor. I typically serve this dahl on its own, but it's delicious topped with roasted veggies.

1. Place the lentils in a pot and cover with the water. Add the turmeric and salt and bring to a boil. Reduce to a simmer and cook, stirring occasionally, until the lentils have broken down and the mixture is soft and soupy, 15 to 20 minutes. Top up with water if necessary.

2. **For the tarka:** Meanwhile, heat the avocado oil in a nonstick pan over medium heat. Add the coriander, cumin, fennel, and mustard seeds and toast, stirring frequently, for about 2 minutes, until fragrant. Add the onion, garlic, ginger, and cilantro and cook until softened, about 8 minutes. Add the tomato and cook another 5 minutes. Season with salt.

3. To serve the dahl, stir the tarka into the lentils. Divide among bowls and top each with cilantro and a lime wedge.

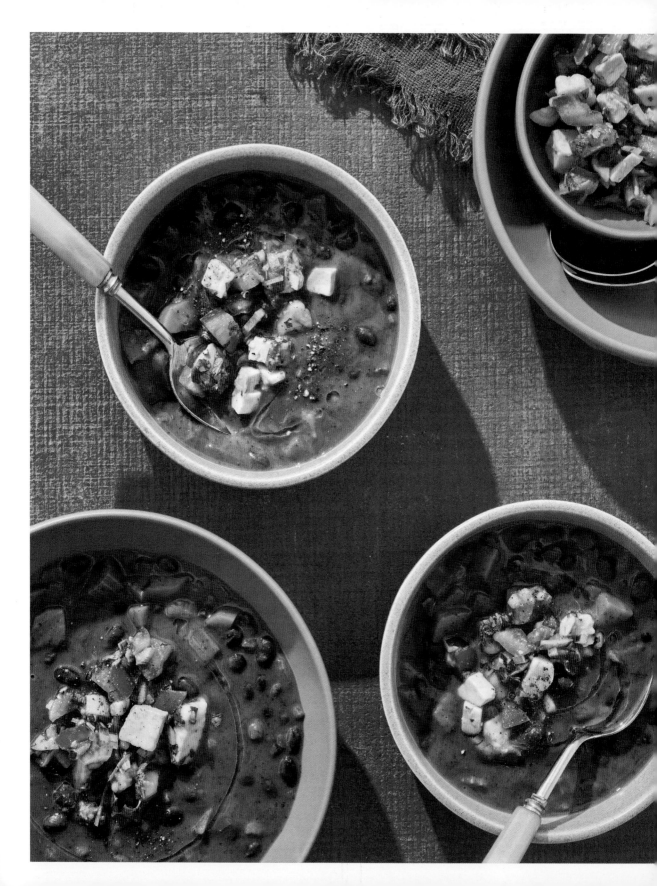

Black Bean Soup
with Tomato Salsa

Serves: 4

Prep Time: 15 minutes
Cook Time: 40 minutes

Soup

1 tablespoon extra-virgin olive oil

1 yellow onion, finely chopped

1 medium carrot, peeled and finely chopped

2 stalks celery, finely chopped

1 jalapeño, seeded and finely chopped

2 garlic cloves, minced

1 tablespoon tomato paste

2 (19-ounce) cans black beans, drained and rinsed

1 tablespoon red wine vinegar

1 teaspoon ground cumin

1 teaspoon smoked paprika

½ teaspoon dried oregano

4 cups vegetable stock

1 teaspoon kosher salt, plus more to taste

½ teaspoon freshly ground black pepper

Salsa

1 avocado, pitted, peeled, and cubed

1 medium tomato, diced

¼ cup finely chopped red onion

½ cup roughly chopped fresh cilantro leaves

1 tablespoon lime juice

½ teaspoon kosher salt

Most black bean soups are stodgy and thick and take hours to cook because of the dried beans. This version is lighter and made with canned beans, which are equally as nutritious but cook in a fraction of the time. Black beans are a highly digestible plant-protein containing fiber and the polyphenol anthocyanin, which are both good for heart health. Laced with cumin and with a kick from smoked paprika, this black bean and vegetable soup makes a delicious weeknight meal.

1. **For the soup:** Heat the olive oil in a large pot over medium heat. Add the onion, carrot, and celery and sauté until softened, about 5 minutes. Add the jalapeño and garlic and cook for 1 minute. Stir in the tomato paste. Add the beans, vinegar, cumin, paprika, and oregano. Add the stock and season with salt and pepper. Bring to a boil, then reduce to a simmer and cook, uncovered, for 25 to 30 minutes.

2. **For the salsa:** Meanwhile, in a medium bowl, mix all the ingredients and set the salsa aside.

3. Using a blender or immersion blender, puree one-third of the soup. Adjust seasoning if needed. Divide the soup among bowls and top with salsa.

Roasted Cauliflower Soup

Serves: 4

Prep Time: 10 minutes

Cook Time: 50 minutes

5 tablespoons extra-virgin
olive oil

1 teaspoon grated lemon zest

1 teaspoon ground cumin

½ teaspoon ground coriander

1 large head cauliflower,
stemmed and broken into florets

1½ teaspoons kosher salt

1 teaspoon freshly ground
black pepper

2 large shallots, roughly chopped

3 small garlic cloves, thinly sliced

1 (15.5-ounce) can cannellini
beans, drained and rinsed

4 to 5 cups vegetable stock

1½ cups water

2 tablespoons finely chopped
fresh chives, for garnish

⅓ cup toasted pumpkin seeds,
for garnish

Roasting cauliflower transforms the cruciferous vegetable into a flavor powerhouse. The key is getting the florets nice and golden as the edges begin to caramelize, which yields big bold flavor for soup. We've added cannellini beans to increase the protein in this low-carbohydrate soup—and with its super creamy consistency, you would never guess it's dairy-free. This is a great make-ahead soup that freezes well.

1. Preheat the oven to 425°F and line a baking sheet with parchment paper.

2. In a large bowl, stir together 3 tablespoons of the olive oil, the lemon zest, cumin, and coriander. Add the cauliflower florets with ½ teaspoon of the salt and ½ teaspoon of the black pepper and toss to coat. Transfer to the baking sheet and roast for 30 to 35 minutes, stirring halfway, until the cauliflower is golden and slightly charred.

3. Meanwhile, in a large pot, heat the remaining 2 tablespoons olive oil over medium heat. Add the shallots and sauté until softened, about 5 minutes. Add the garlic and cook for another minute, until fragrant. Add the beans, vegetable stock, and water. Season with the remaining 1 teaspoon salt and ½ teaspoon pepper. Bring to a boil, then remove from the heat and set aside until the cauliflower is done.

4. Add the roasted cauliflower to the pot and bring to a boil. Reduce the heat to low, cover, and simmer for 10 minutes. Remove from the heat and puree with an immersion blender in the pot, or in small batches in a blender, until smooth. Divide among bowls and garnish with fresh chives and toasted pumpkin seeds.

Chipotle Bison Chili

Serves: 6

Prep Time: 15 minutes

Cook Time: 2 hours

1 tablespoon extra-virgin olive oil

1 pound ground grass-fed bison

1 yellow onion, diced

2 garlic cloves, minced

1½ teaspoons kosher salt, plus more to taste

½ teaspoon freshly ground black pepper

10 ounces cremini mushrooms, roughly chopped

2 tablespoons chopped chipotle pepper in adobo

1 tablespoon chili powder

1 teaspoon dried oregano

1 teaspoon ground cumin

1 cup dark stout beer

1 tablespoon red wine vinegar

2 teaspoons Worcestershire sauce

1 (28-ounce) can diced tomatoes

2 to 3 cups chicken stock

1 (15.5-ounce) can pinto beans, drained and rinsed

½ cup goat or sheep's milk yogurt, for serving

Although not the most common ingredient, bison is an extremely nutritious source of low-fat protein. It's loaded with vitamins B_{12} and B_6, zinc, iron, and two essential fatty acids, omega-3 and omega-6. Talk about a powerhouse of nutrition that will boost your energy and increase endurance! I love ground bison in this chili because of its mild flavor and adaptability to all the warming spices. The slow-cooked chili is a great make-ahead meal as it becomes richer and more complex if you give it a day or so to sit before serving.

1. Heat the olive oil in a heavy large pot over medium heat. Add the bison and sauté, breaking up the meat with a spoon, until browned, about 5 minutes. Add the onion and garlic and continue cooking until the onions are translucent, 6 to 8 minutes. Season with the salt and pepper.

2. Add the mushrooms and cook for another 5 minutes, until they begin to sweat. Add the chipotles, chili powder, oregano, and cumin and stir until fragrant. Deglaze the pot with the beer and vinegar and cook for 2 to 3 minutes, until the liquid has reduced by half.

3. Season with Worcestershire sauce then add the diced tomatoes and chicken stock. Bring to a boil, then simmer until thickened, about 1 hour 30 minutes. Add the beans and continue cooking for another 5 minutes, until heated through.

4. Serve the chili in bowls with a good dollop of yogurt.

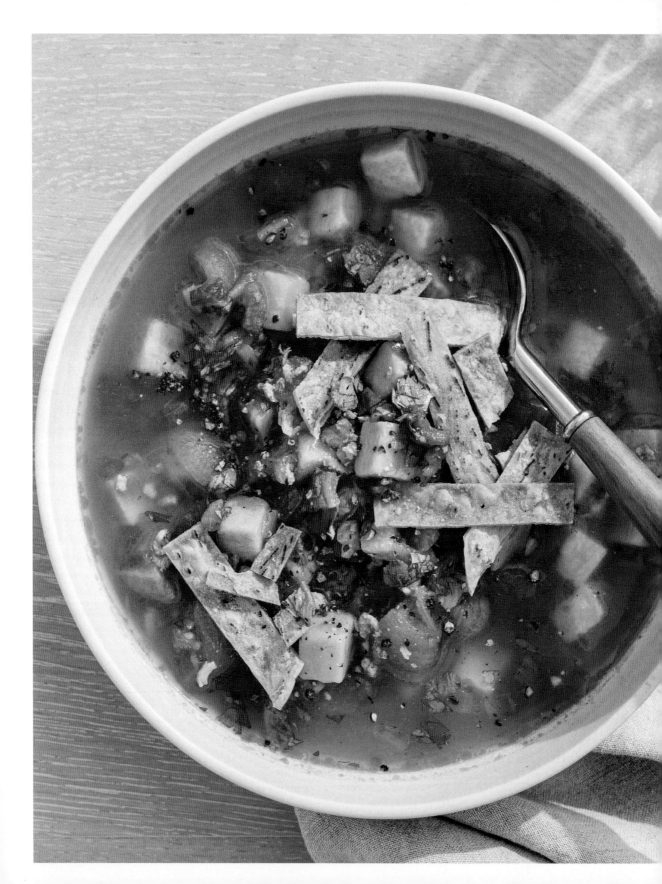

Chicken Tortilla Soup

Serves: 6

Prep Time: 15 minutes

Cook Time: 1 hour

5 large tomatoes, halved

4 large jalapeños, halved

5 garlic cloves, unpeeled

2 tablespoons extra-virgin olive oil

1 pound ground pasture-raised chicken

1 yellow onion, diced

1 small sweet potato, peeled and cubed

1 red bell pepper, stemmed, seeded, and diced

1 tablespoon tomato paste

1 teaspoon ground cumin

½ teaspoon onion powder

½ teaspoon dried oregano

4 cups chicken stock

1 teaspoon kosher salt

½ teaspoon freshly ground black pepper

Tortilla Chips

4 corn tortillas, halved, then cut into strips

1 tablespoon extra-virgin olive oil

Jalapeño Salsa

2 tablespoons lime juice

½ cup loosely packed fresh cilantro leaves, roughly chopped

½ teaspoon kosher salt

This recipe, a riff on tortilla soup, uses a technique of broiling tomatoes and jalapeño peppers to create the smokiness that would traditionally come from an open fire. I've added ground chicken for lean protein with anti-inflammatory effects and a jalapeño salsa for some extra spice.

1. Preheat the broiler to high. Line a baking sheet with tin foil. Arrange the tomatoes and jalapeños cut side up on the sheet and scatter the garlic cloves around. Broil for 10 minutes, checking every couple of minutes to rotate the pan if needed, until the vegetables are charred. Remove and set aside to cool slightly.

2. Roughly chop the broiled tomatoes and place in a bowl. Squeeze the garlic from the skins into the bowl with the tomatoes. Remove and discard the charred skins and seeds from the jalapeños and roughly chop the flesh; set aside in a separate bowl.

3. Heat the olive oil in a large pot over medium heat. Add the ground chicken and cook, breaking up the meat with a wooden spoon, for 5 minutes, until golden and cooked through. Add the onion and cook until soft, 6 to 8 minutes. Add 1 tablespoon of chopped jalapeños (set aside the rest for the salsa).

4. Stir in the sweet potato and red pepper and cook for 5 minutes, until they begin to soften. Add the tomato paste, cumin, onion powder, and oregano, stirring until fragrant. Add the chicken stock and broiled tomato mixture. Season with the salt and pepper and bring to a boil. Reduce to a simmer and cook for 30 minutes, partially covered.

5. For the tortilla chips: Meanwhile, preheat the oven to 400°F. Line a baking sheet with parchment paper. Toss the tortilla strips with olive oil and transfer to a single layer on the baking sheet. Bake for 8 to 10 minutes, flipping halfway, until golden.

6. For the jalapeño salsa: In a small bowl, toss the remaining chopped jalapeños with the lime juice and cilantro. Season with salt to taste.

7. To serve, ladle the soup into bowls and top each with a spoonful of the jalapeño salsa and a few crispy tortilla chips.

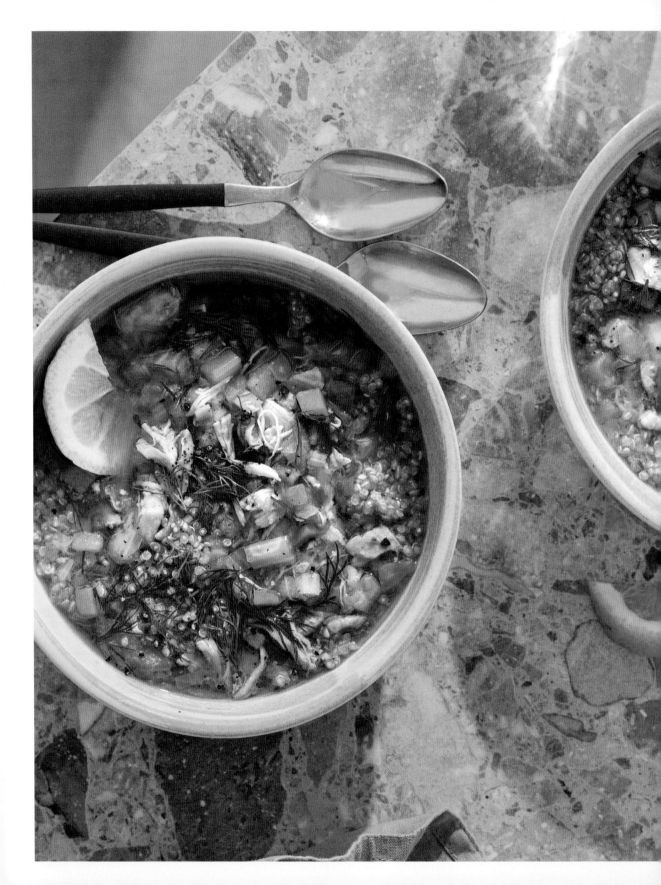

Lemony Dill, Chicken, and Quinoa Soup

Serves: 4 to 6

Prep Time: 20 minutes

Cook Time: 1 hour

1 tablespoon extra-virgin olive oil

6 to 8 bone-in skin-on pasture-raised chicken thighs

1 large leek, quartered and thinly sliced

1 small fennel bulb, cored and diced

1 medium carrot, peeled and diced

2 stalks celery, diced

1 tablespoon tomato paste

1 strip lemon zest

4 cups chicken stock, plus more if needed

1 small bunch fresh flat-leaf parsley, plus ¼ cup finely chopped

1 small bunch fresh dill, plus ¼ cup finely chopped

4 sprigs fresh thyme

1 teaspoon kosher salt

1 teaspoon freshly ground black pepper

1 cup quinoa

1½ cups water

1 lemon, cut into wedges, for serving

This speedier version of chicken soup, using bone-in chicken thighs, not only cuts down on time, but adds a significant amount of flavor and nutrition. Collagen, a connective tissue, breaks down into gelatin and other health-promoting, anti-aging amino acids when cooked and creates a delicious chicken bone broth. Full of fresh herbs, lemon, and fragrant fennel, this chicken soup is one you will want to make time and time again.

1. Heat the olive oil in a large heavy pot over medium heat. Add the chicken and brown for 4 minutes per side, until the skin is crisp and golden. Remove and set aside.

2. Carefully wipe out most of the oil from the pot, leaving only a tablespoon. Add the leek, fennel, carrot, and celery and cook for 6 to 8 minutes, until softened. Stir in the tomato paste and lemon zest, then pour in the chicken stock. Add the chicken thighs, adding more stock or water if necessary to just cover them. With kitchen twine, tie the parsley, dill, and thyme bunches together. Add the bundle to the soup along with the salt and pepper. Bring the soup to a boil, reduce to a simmer, partially cover, and simmer for 40 minutes.

3. Meanwhile, place the quinoa and water in a small pot. Bring to a boil, then reduce to a simmer, cover, and cook for 12 minutes, until all the liquid is absorbed. Remove from the heat, fluff with a fork, and set aside.

4. Remove the chicken thighs from the pot and let cool slightly, then pull the meat from the bones; discard the skin and bones. Add the shredded meat back to the soup. Fish out the herb bundle and discard. Stir in the chopped parsley and dill.

5. To serve, add scoops of quinoa to bowls. Ladle in the soup and serve with lemon wedges for squeezing over the top.

Kombu and Mushroom Broth

Serves: 4

Prep Time: 15 minutes

Cook Time: 40 minutes

3 (5x1-inch) strips kombu

8 cups water

4 ounces dried shiitake mushrooms, rinsed

4 scallions, whites cut into 1-inch pieces, greens sliced and reserved for optional garnish

1 tablespoon finely grated fresh ginger

3 tablespoons gluten-free tamari

1 tablespoon mirin

1 teaspoon fish sauce (optional)

6 ounces fresh shiitake mushrooms, sliced

1 carrot, peeled and sliced

2 cups packed baby spinach

1 (8-ounce) package soft organic tofu, cut into cubes

¼ cup natto

The base of this superfood immunity soup is dashi, a delicate stock made from dried kombu seaweed. Kombu is not only full of umami, it also contains iodine, which is important for thyroid function. The broth is fortified with fresh shiitakes, spinach, and tofu, then topped with natto, a Japanese fermented soybean product filled with probiotics. Although it has a slimy texture, once stirred into the broth natto adds a delicious, complex flavor.

1.   **For the dashi:** Combine the kombu and water in a pot and bring to a boil. Remove from the heat and let sit for 10 minutes. Discard the kombu. Add the dried shiitakes and scallion whites. Bring to a boil, reduce the heat, and simmer for 30 minutes, uncovered. Stir in the ginger, tamari, mirin, and fish sauce, if using. Strain the broth and discard the mushrooms.

2.   **For the soup:** Return the broth to the pot and bring to a simmer. Add the fresh shiitakes and carrot and cook for 6 minutes, until softened. Stir in the spinach and tofu and simmer for about a minute.

3.   Ladle the broth into bowls and top with spoonfuls of natto and reserved scallion greens, if desired.

Harissa Chickpea Stew

Serves: 4 to 6
Prep Time: 15 minutes
Cook Time: 1 hour

1 tablespoon extra-virgin olive oil

1 medium red onion, diced

1 large sweet potato, peeled and cubed

1 large carrot, peeled and cubed

2 garlic cloves, finely chopped

1 tablespoon finely chopped fresh ginger

½ cup tightly packed fresh cilantro, stems finely chopped, leaves reserved for garnish

1 teaspoon kosher salt, plus more to taste

½ teaspoon freshly ground black pepper

2 tablespoons harissa

2 teaspoons ground cumin

1 cinnamon stick

2 (28-ounce) cans diced tomatoes

4 cups vegetable stock

1 (15.5-ounce) can chickpeas, drained and rinsed

⅓ cup dried apricots, roughly chopped

3 cups baby spinach

Comforting and simple to make, this is a great vegetarian one-pot meal you can batch prepare and freeze to have on hand when life gets busy. Harissa, a North African spiced paste, adds a rich layer of flavor and heat to an otherwise simple vegetable stew. Protein-rich chickpeas and antioxidant-rich baby spinach, which contain essential anti-aging vitamins beta-carotene and lutein, make this a nutrient-dense, satisfying stew for those cooler nights.

1. Heat the olive oil in a large pot over medium heat. Add the onion and sauté until translucent, about 6 minutes. Add the sweet potato and carrot and continue cooking until softened, about 8 minutes. Stir in the garlic, ginger, and cilantro stems and season with the salt and pepper. Add the harissa, cumin, and cinnamon stick and cook for a minute or so, until fragrant. Add the diced tomatoes and stock. Bring to a boil, then reduce to a simmer and cook for 30 minutes. Add the chickpeas and apricots and continue cooking for 10 minutes.

2. Stir in the baby spinach and cook until wilted, about 2 minutes. Season to taste with salt and garnish with reserved cilantro leaves. Serve immediately.

Tip: *This stew can be transformed into a more filling meal by serving with a scoop of cooked brown rice or quinoa.*

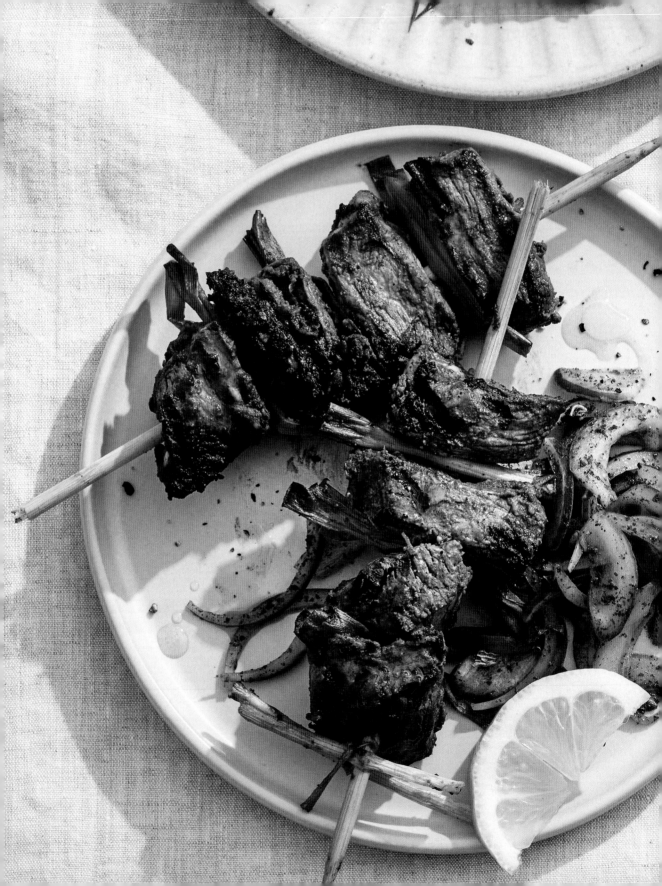

Poultry and Meat

Protein provides us with the building blocks essential for optimal performance and longevity. Our muscle mass decreases as we age, so it's important to include high-quality animal proteins, in moderation, to help maintain and repair our muscles as well as reduce our risk of age-related chronic disease. These mouth-watering recipes, like Smoky Turkish Beef Kebabs (page 112), Berbere Chicken with Tahini (page 109), and Braised Pomegranate Lamb Shanks (page 116), will add plenty of protein, beneficial nutrients, and new and exciting flavors to your dinner table.

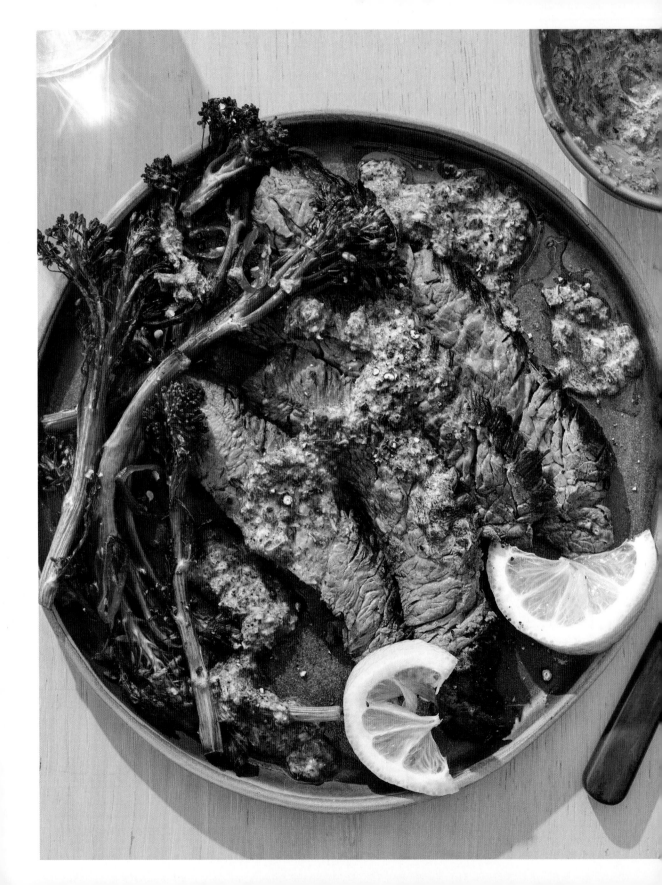

Balsamic Marinated Steak with Broccolini

Serves: 4 to 6
Prep Time: 10 minutes
plus 30 minutes marinating
Cook Time: 30 minutes

Steak

2 tablespoons extra-virgin
olive oil

¼ cup balsamic vinegar

2 tablespoons apple cider
vinegar

5 garlic cloves, smashed

1 teaspoon kosher salt

½ teaspoon freshly ground
black pepper

1½ pounds grass-fed
skirt steak

Broccolini

1 pound broccolini, trimmed
and halved lengthwise

¼ cup extra-virgin olive oil

3 garlic cloves, smashed

1 long red chile, sliced

1 lemon, cut into wedges

2 tablespoons avocado oil,
for grilling

Salsa Verde (page 205),
for serving

Skirt steak is an affordable marbled cut that tastes even better when marinated. (If you can't find skirt steak, use another quick cooking cut like hanger or strip loin.) The key to delicious skirt steak is to cook it on a hot grill to sear the outside and then slice the meat against the grain once it's cooked and rested. Along with simple roasted broccolini and my zesty salsa verde, this is a tasty meal that could easily be served midweek or for entertaining.

1. **To marinate the steak:** Combine the olive oil, balsamic vinegar, cider vinegar, garlic, salt, and pepper in a sealable bag. Add the steak and rub the mixture into the meat. Seal the bag and marinate at room temperature for 30 minutes, or in the refrigerator overnight.

2. **For the broccolini:** Preheat the oven to 425°F. In a medium bowl, toss the broccolini with the olive oil, garlic, chile, and lemon wedges until well coated. Transfer to a baking sheet and roast for 15 to 20 minutes, until the broccolini is bright green and crispy at the edges.

3. Preheat the grill to 450°F (or heat a cast-iron pan on the stovetop over high heat). Oil the grill grates with the avocado oil. Grill the steak for 3 to 5 minutes per side depending on the thickness of the steak, until an internal temperature reads 130°F for medium-rare. Remove and rest for at least 10 minutes.

4. Slice the steak into strips against the grain and serve with the broccolini and Salsa Verde.

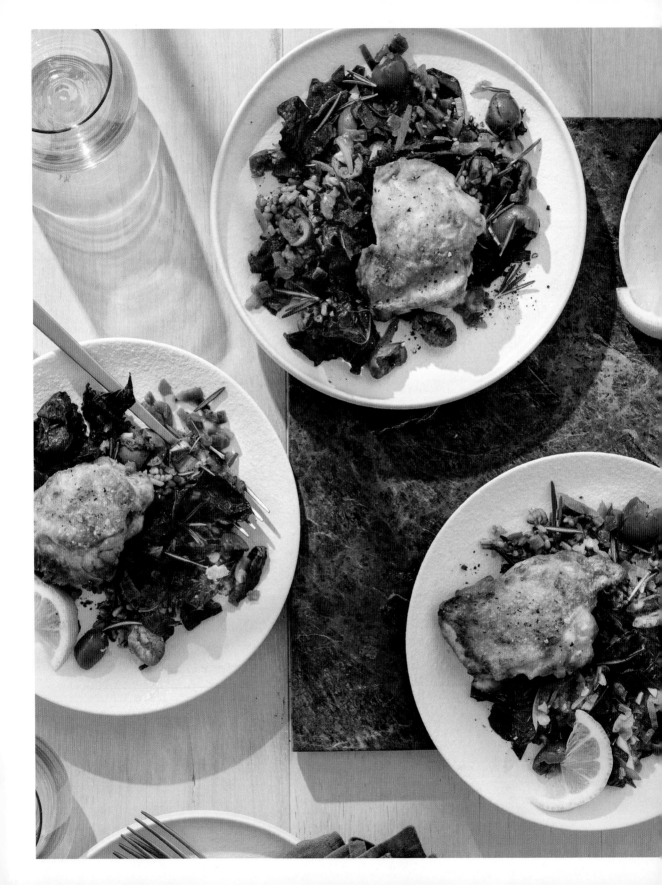

Chicken with Kale
and Preserved Lemon

Serves: 4 to 6

Prep Time: 15 minutes

Cook Time: 40 minutes

1 cup brown basmati rice

2 cups water

8 bone-in skin-on pasture-raised chicken thighs

1½ teaspoons kosher salt

½ teaspoon ground black pepper

1 tablespoon extra-virgin olive oil

1 red onion, diced

3 garlic cloves, thinly sliced

1 heaping tablespoon finely chopped preserved lemon, seeds removed

1 bunch Tuscan kale, deveined and sliced

⅔ cup green Castelvetrano olives, pitted and roughly chopped

1 fresh rosemary sprig

1 cup chicken stock

¼ cup lemon juice

I love the simplicity of a one-pan meal. Juicy roasted chicken thighs with briny olives and a lemony, umami kick from preserved lemon go so well with braised kale, which is packed with folate and phytonutrients. The preserved lemon shouldn't be skipped as it adds a bright unique flavor you can't get from regular lemons. But if you can't find preserved lemons, add a squeeze of fresh lemon juice at the end.

1. Combine the rice and water in a pot and add a pinch of salt. Bring to a boil, then reduce to a simmer and cook, covered, for 25 to 30 minutes, until the water is absorbed and the rice is soft.

2. Meanwhile, cook the chicken: Season the chicken liberally with 1 teaspoon of the salt and the black pepper. In a large heavy skillet (preferably cast iron) fitted with a lid, heat the olive oil over medium heat. Working in batches, add the chicken thighs skin-side down and cook for 5 to 7 minutes, until deep golden brown. Flip and continue cooking for another 3 to 4 minutes. Transfer the chicken to a plate and set aside.

3. Wipe out the excess oil in the pan, leaving about 2 tablespoons. Reduce the heat to low, add the onion, and cook, scraping up all the brown bits from the pan with a wooden spoon, until the onion is softened and translucent, about 3 minutes. Add the garlic and preserved lemon and cook until fragrant, about 1 minute. Season with the remaining ½ teaspoon salt.

4. Preheat the broiler to high.

5. Add the kale to the pan and cook until wilted slightly, about 2 minutes. Return the chicken to the pan and scatter the olives and rosemary sprig over. Pour the chicken stock and lemon juice into the pan and bring to a boil. Cover and cook for about 10 minutes.

6. Remove the lid, transfer the pan to the oven, and broil for 1 to 2 minutes, until the chicken skin is crispy.

7. To serve, add a scoop of brown rice to each plate. Top with kale, chicken, and olives. Use a spoon to drizzle any pan juices over the meat.

Spice-Roasted Leg of Lamb

Serves: 6 to 8

Prep Time: 10 minutes

Cook Time: 1 hour 30 minutes

1 (6-pound) grass-fed leg of lamb, shank bone removed

6 garlic cloves, finely grated

Grated zest of 1 lemon

1 tablespoon finely chopped rosemary leaves

1 tablespoon toasted coriander seeds

2 teaspoons toasted cumin seeds

1 tablespoon kosher salt

½ teaspoon freshly ground black pepper

½ cup (1 stick) unsalted grass-fed butter, softened to room temperature

1 lemon, halved

2 cups dry white wine

Pistachio Mint Pesto (page 201), for serving

A leg of lamb is a meal to impress, and although it sounds intimidating, it's one of the simpler cuts to cook well. Lamb is one of the best meat sources of iron as well as vitamins B_{12} and B_6, which aid in a healthy nervous system and metabolism. What I love about this recipe is the aromatic spice rub, which adds so much flavor. Paired with my Pistachio Mint Pesto, this is an impressive recipe perfect for entertaining.

1. Remove the lamb from the fridge 1 hour prior to cooking to come to room temperature.

2. Preheat the oven to 425°F. Using a small knife, make small incisions about 2 inches deep all over the lamb.

3. In a food processor (or with a mortar and pestle), combine the garlic, lemon zest, rosemary, coriander seeds, cumin seeds, salt, and pepper and blend until almost smooth. Add the butter and pulse until it comes together into a thick paste. Using your hands, rub the paste all over the lamb, pressing it into the incisions.

4. Place the lamb on a rack in a roasting pan, fat side up. Squeeze the lemon juice all over and pour the wine around the lamb. Roast for 15 minutes, then reduce the heat to 350°F. Roast for 60 to 90 minutes, basting every 20 minutes or so and adding more wine if needed, until the internal temperature reaches 150°F.

5. Tent with foil and let rest for at least 20 minutes before carving. Serve with the Pistachio Mint Pesto.

Bison Meatballs with Braised White Beans

Serves: 4

Prep Time: 15 minutes

Cook Time: 20 minutes

Meatballs

1 egg

1 tablespoon extra-virgin olive oil

½ cup almond flour

2 tablespoons finely chopped fresh basil

2 tablespoons finely chopped fresh dill, plus more for garnish

1 teaspoon kosher salt

½ teaspoon freshly ground black pepper

1 pound grass-fed ground bison

Beans

2 tablespoons extra-virgin olive oil

1 small fennel bulb, cored and finely chopped

1 small yellow onion, finely chopped

3 garlic cloves, minced

¼ teaspoon red pepper flakes

1 pound cherry tomatoes

1 (15.5-ounce) can cannellini beans, drained and rinsed

2 cups vegetable or chicken stock

1 teaspoon kosher salt, plus more to taste

½ teaspoon ground black pepper

1 teaspoon grated lemon zest

1 tablespoon lemon juice

Meatballs are a great make-ahead meal, perfect for that post-work dinner when you're short on time. This healthy, protein-rich recipe is made with ground bison, a leaner, omega-3-rich alternative to beef. Roasting the meatballs in the oven cuts down on cleanup and gives you the perfect amount of time to braise the beans. The beans are loaded with fresh, sweet cherry tomatoes, which provide ample nutrition. When cooked, tomatoes release higher amounts of lycopene, a cancer-fighting antioxidant. These beans are great on their own and can easily be doubled if you're looking for a simple recipe to meal prep.

1. Preheat the oven to 400°F and set the oven rack in the middle. Line a baking sheet with parchment paper.

2. For the meatballs: In a large bowl, whisk together the egg and olive oil. Add the almond flour and mix until it is no longer dry. Add the basil, dill, salt, and pepper, mixing well. Add half the bison meat, working the herb mixture into the meat with your hands. Then mix in the remaining meat, being careful not to overwork. Form the meat into twelve balls and set them on the baking sheet. Bake for 15 minutes, until they are cooked through.

3. For the beans: Meanwhile, heat the olive oil in a large nonstick pan over medium heat. Add the fennel and onion and cook for 4 minutes, until softened. Add the garlic and red pepper flakes and cook until fragrant, about 1 minute. Add the cherry tomatoes and cook for 5 minutes, until the skins soften.

4. Stir in the beans, stock, salt, and pepper. Bring to a boil, then reduce to a simmer. Use the back of a wooden spoon to gently mash some of the beans, then cook for about 8 minutes, until the liquid has reduced and the mixture has thickened. Stir in the lemon zest and juice, to taste.

5. To serve, scoop some of the braised beans onto plates and top with meatballs. Sprinkle with the remaining dill.

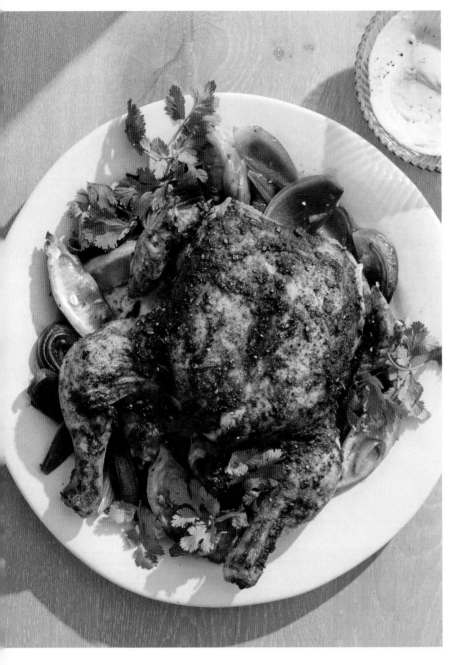

Serves: 4
Prep Time: 15 minutes
Cook Time: 1 hour 15 minutes

Berbere Spice Mix

1 tablespoon ground cumin

1 tablespoon smoked paprika

1 teaspoon ground fenugreek
(or ½ teaspoon ground yellow
mustard seeds)

1 teaspoon ground coriander

½ teaspoon ground ginger

½ teaspoon freshly ground
black pepper

¼ teaspoon ground cinnamon

¼ teaspoon cayenne pepper,
or to taste

Chicken

2 garlic cloves, minced

1 teaspoon kosher salt

3 tablespoons extra-virgin
olive oil

1 (4-pound) pasture-raised
chicken, spatchcocked (see Tips)

2 red onions, cut into 1-inch
wedges

2 lemons, quartered

½ teaspoon freshly ground
black pepper

Berbere Chicken with Tahini

Tahini Sauce

⅓ cup tahini

2 to 4 tablespoons lemon juice

1 garlic clove, grated

½ teaspoon ground cumin

½ teaspoon kosher salt

¼ teaspoon freshly ground black pepper

¼ cup fresh cilantro leaves, for garnish

Berbere is a versatile Ethiopian spice blend made with cumin, cinnamon, and fenugreek that pairs well with chicken. I especially love how this whole roasted chicken comes together in one pan, with the flavorful juices of the roast trickling down onto the vegetables underneath. By flattening, or spatchcocking the bird, you cut down slightly on the cooking time, but more importantly you get wonderfully juicy meat and crispy skin all over. This recipe pairs well with my Caramelized Carrots with Lime Yogurt (page 151).

1. Preheat the oven to 425°F.

2. **For the spice mix:** In a small jar fitted with a lid, add all the ingredients and shake well until combined.

3. **For the chicken:** Place the minced garlic on the cutting board and sprinkle with the salt. Using the flat part of your knife blade, press the salt into the garlic continuously until a paste forms. Transfer the garlic to a small bowl and mix in 1 heaping tablespoon of the berbere spice mix and 1 tablespoon of the olive oil. Rub the paste generously over the chicken.

4. In a large cast-iron pan, add the onions and lemon wedges. Drizzle with the remaining 2 tablespoons olive oil and mix well. Place the chicken on top and sprinkle the pepper all over. Roast in the oven for 15 minutes. Reduce the heat to 350°F and continue roasting for 1 hour, or until the internal temperature of the chicken reaches 165°F.

5. **For the tahini sauce:** In a small bowl, combine the tahini, 2 tablespoons lemon juice, the garlic, cumin, salt, and pepper. Whisk until smooth, adding ¼ cup water and more lemon juice if necessary for seasoning and desired consistency.

6. Transfer the chicken to a platter along with the onions and lemon wedges. Drizzle with the tahini sauce, sprinkle with cilantro leaves, and serve.

Tip: To spatchcock a chicken, use kitchen shears to cut on either side of the backbone and remove it completely. Flip the bird over and push down to flatten it. You can also ask your butcher to do this.

Tip: Store remaining berbere spice mix in an airtight container in your pantry. Use it when roasting vegetables or marinating meat.

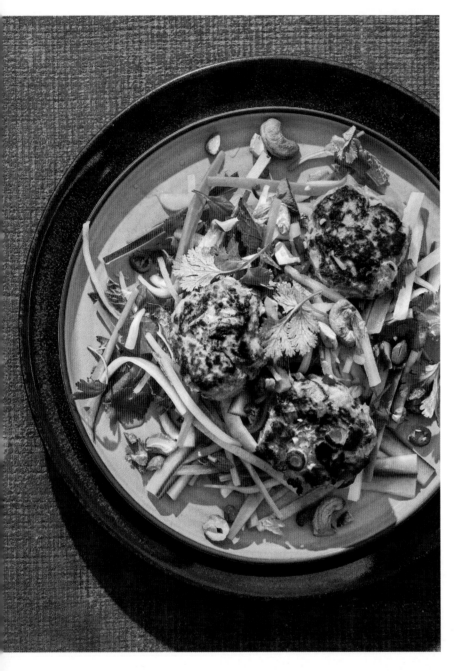

Serves: 4
Prep Time: 30 minutes
Cook Time: 20 minutes

Patties

1 pound pasture-raised ground turkey

1 lemongrass stalk, outer layer removed, bulb and light green part minced

1 small zucchini, grated and gently squeezed to remove excess moisture

⅓ cup thinly sliced scallions

2 tablespoons finely chopped fresh cilantro

2 garlic cloves, grated

1 tablespoon fish sauce

2 tablespoons avocado oil

Dressing

3 tablespoons fish sauce

3 tablespoons lime juice

2 tablespoons rice wine vinegar

1 tablespoon maple syrup

1 tablespoon water

1 red Thai chile, seeded and finely chopped (optional)

1 garlic clove, minced

Vietnamese Turkey Bun Cha

Salad

2 medium carrots, peeled and julienned

½ English cucumber, julienned

¼ large daikon radish, peeled and julienned

1 cup bean sprouts

1 cup roughly chopped fresh cilantro leaves, plus more for garnish

1 cup roughly chopped fresh mint leaves, plus more for garnish

⅓ cup chopped toasted cashews, plus more for garnish

2 limes, cut into wedges, for serving

These Vietnamese turkey patties are a great make-ahead protein as you can enjoy them cold with the crunchy salad or on their own. Ground turkey is a delicious, affordable lean protein and an excellent source of vitamin B_{12} and niacin, both of which can help regulate your digestive and nervous systems. I've added even more nutrition with zucchini, which is rich in vitamin C. This crispy crunchy bun cha is the perfect midweek meal.

1. Preheat the oven to 400°F and line a baking sheet with parchment paper.

2. **For the patties:** In a large bowl, combine all the patty ingredients except the avocado oil with your hands, being careful not to overwork. Divide into twelve portions and shape into patties. Refrigerate for 10 minutes.

3. Heat 1 tablespoon of the avocado oil in a large nonstick pan over medium heat. Working in batches, add half the patties and cook for 2 to 3 minutes per side, until golden brown, then transfer to the prepared baking sheet. Allow the pan to cool slightly. Heat the remaining tablespoon oil and continue cooking the patties. Transfer the baking sheet to the oven and bake for 10 minutes, or until the patties reach an internal temperature of 165°F.

4. **For the salad dressing:** In a small bowl, whisk all the ingredients together.

5. **For the salad:** In a large bowl, combine all the ingredients except the lime wedges.

6. To serve, toss the salad with most of the dressing and place in shallow bowls. Top with a couple turkey patties and an extra drizzle of dressing. Sprinkle with additional cilantro, mint leaves, and chopped cashews and serve with lime wedges.

Tip: *These turkey patties make an excellent snack on their own, and they freeze well. Double the batch!*

Smoky Turkish Beef Kebabs

Serves: 4 to 6

Prep Time: 30 minutes

Cook Time: 10 minutes

Kebabs

2 tablespoons extra-virgin olive oil

2 tablespoons grated yellow onion

1 tablespoon tomato puree

4 garlic cloves, grated

1 tablespoon smoked paprika

1 teaspoon ground cumin

1 teaspoon kosher salt

½ teaspoon cayenne pepper

½ teaspoon freshly ground black pepper

2½ pounds grass-fed top sirloin, cut into 1-inch cubes

1 large bunch scallions, cut into 3-inch pieces

Avocado oil, for grilling

Onion Salad

1 red onion, thinly sliced

1 tablespoon extra-virgin olive oil

2 tablespoons lemon juice

2 teaspoons ground sumac

1 teaspoon kosher salt

2 tablespoons finely chopped fresh mint

These kebabs are great for summertime grilling as sirloin is a lean cut that cooks quickly while remaining tender. The skewers are paired with a bright onion salad seasoned with sumac, a lemony, tangy, and slightly acidic spice made from ground berries. Marinate the kebabs overnight for even more flavor, then serve alongside my Spiced Kohlrabi with Pomegranate and Feta (page 154) for a complete meal. You'll need to soak 10 bamboo skewers in water for a few minutes before threading on the kebabs and scallions.

1. **For the kebabs:** In a large bowl, combine the olive oil, onion, tomato puree, garlic, paprika, cumin, salt, cayenne, and black pepper. Add the beef cubes, tossing to coat. Marinate at room temperature for at least 20 minutes, or refrigerate overnight.

2. Thread three or four cubes of meat onto the skewers, alternating them with the scallion pieces.

3. **For the onion salad:** Combine the onion, olive oil, lemon juice, sumac, and salt in a small bowl. Use your hands to gently massage the onions, mixing everything well, then stir in the mint.

4. Preheat the grill to 450°F or heat a grill pan over medium-high heat. Lightly oil the grill with the avocado oil. Grill the skewers for 4 to 5 minutes per side, until the beef is cooked through and the scallions are charred. Serve the skewers with the onion salad on the side.

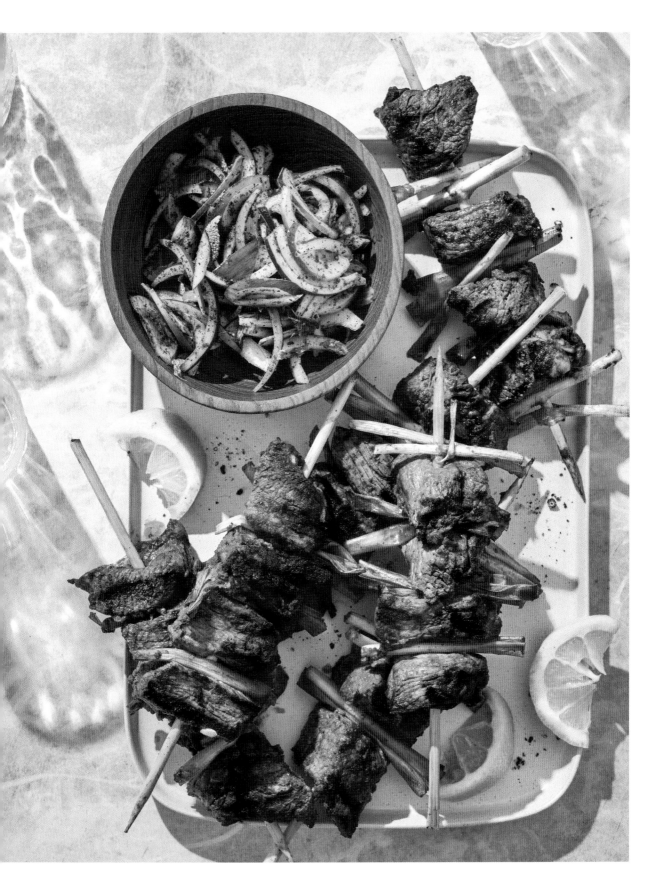

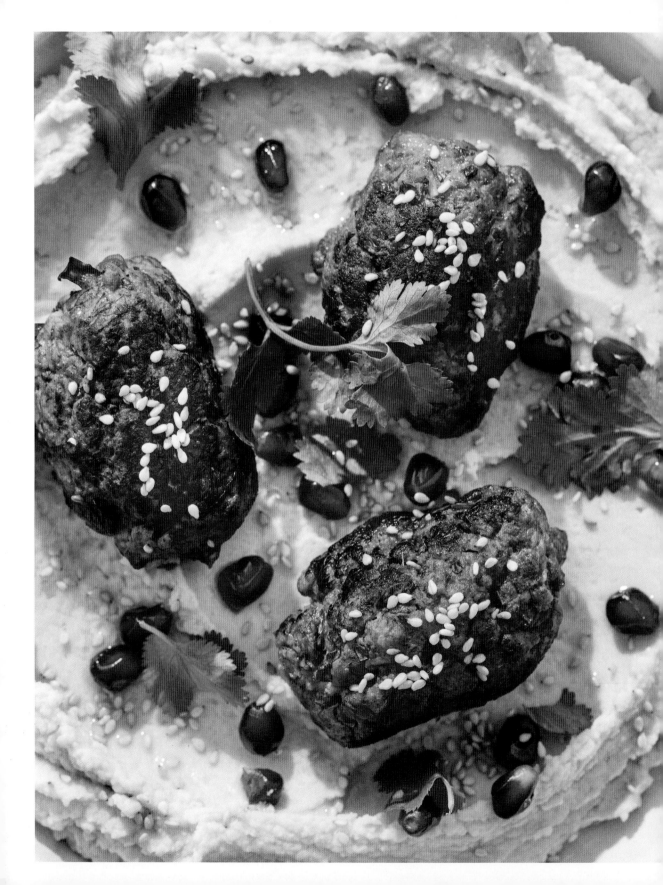

Beef Kofte with Hummus

Serves: 4

Prep Time: 20 minutes

Cook Time: 15 minutes

Kofte

1 pound grass-fed lean ground beef

½ cup grated yellow onion

¼ cup finely chopped fresh flat-leaf parsley

¼ cup finely chopped fresh cilantro

2 garlic cloves, grated

2 teaspoons ground cumin

2 teaspoons sweet paprika

1 teaspoon coriander seeds, toasted and ground

1 teaspoon ground cinnamon

1½ teaspoons kosher salt

1 tablespoon avocado oil

Hummus

1 (15.5-ounce) can chickpeas, drained and rinsed

1 small garlic clove, peeled

¼ cup lemon juice

2 tablespoons tahini

1 teaspoon kosher salt

5 tablespoons ice water

¼ cup toasted sesame seeds, for garnish

½ cup fresh cilantro leaves, for garnish

¼ cup pomegranate seeds, for garnish

These beef kofte, although a simplified version of traditional kofte, have big, bold aromatic flavors. After a quick sear to caramelize, they simply bake in the oven for an easy weeknight dinner. The key is to make sure you don't overwork the ground beef, which would ultimately yield tough kofte. I love to pair them with homemade hummus, which is easy to make and healthier than store-bought versions. Loaded with both plant and meat protein, this is a perfect meal served alongside some steamed greens.

1. **For the kofte:** In a large bowl, combine all the ingredients except the avocado oil, then use your hands to mix well, being careful not to overwork. Divide the mixture into twelve portions, then gently shape into logs. Refrigerate for 10 minutes.

2. Preheat the oven to 400°F and line a baking sheet with parchment paper.

3. Heat the avocado oil in a nonstick pan over medium heat. Add the kofte and brown all over, 1 to 2 minutes. Transfer to the baking sheet and bake for 8 to 10 minutes, until the beef is cooked through with an internal temperature of 160°F.

4. **For the hummus:** Meanwhile, in a food processor, combine the chickpeas and garlic. Pulse a few times then add the lemon juice, tahini, and salt. With the motor running, gradually add the ice water. Leave the motor running for at least 5 minutes for extra smooth and creamy hummus. Transfer to a bowl.

5. To serve, spread a couple tablespoons of hummus on each plate. Top with a few kofte and sprinkle with sesame seeds, cilantro leaves, and pomegranate seeds.

Braised Pomegranate Lamb Shanks

Serves: 4 to 6

Prep Time: 15 minutes

Cook Time: 3 hours

Lamb Shanks

6 grass-fed lamb shanks

2 teaspoons kosher salt,
plus more to taste

1 teaspoon freshly ground
black pepper, plus more to taste

2 tablespoons avocado oil

3 large shallots, halved

6 garlic cloves, smashed

4 sprigs fresh thyme

2 cups dry red wine

2 cups pomegranate juice

1 cup vegetable or chicken stock,
plus more if needed

1 teaspoon whole black
peppercorns

2 tablespoons arrowroot powder
mixed with 2 tablespoons water
(optional)

Pomegranate Gremolata

½ cup pomegranate seeds

½ cup finely chopped fresh
flat-leaf parsley

1 teaspoon grated lemon zest

1 tablespoon lemon juice

1 garlic clove, finely chopped

1 tablespoon extra-virgin olive oil

½ teaspoon kosher salt

Pinch of freshly ground
black pepper

Bone-in lamb shanks are perfect for braising in a combination of red wine and sweet pomegranate juice. The meat becomes tender after slow cooking, and it tastes even better if made a few days ahead and reheated on the stove (see Tip). The rich flavors of the lamb balance nicely with the bright, citrusy pomegranate gremolata served on top. Pomegranate is a longevity superfood, containing polyphenols that produce a unique compound in the gut, called Urolithin A, that can help protect your body from aging.

1. **For the lamb shanks:** Preheat the oven to 325°F. Season the lamb shanks with 1 teaspoon of the salt and the black pepper.

2. Heat the avocado oil in a large Dutch oven or other ovenproof pot over medium heat. Working in batches, sear the shanks on all sides until golden brown, 7 to 8 minutes. Set aside on a rimmed plate.

3. Remove the pot from the heat and use the residual heat to cook the shallots until golden all over, about 3 minutes. Add the garlic and thyme and stir for a minute or so until fragrant.

4. Place the pot back on the burner and turn the heat to medium-high. Add the wine and deglaze the pot, scraping up any bits. Boil for 3 minutes, then add the pomegranate juice, stock, peppercorns, and remaining 1 teaspoon salt. Return the shanks to the pot and arrange them so they are almost all covered with liquid, adding more stock if needed. Soak a piece of parchment paper under running water, then crumple it up. Lay it directly on top of the lamb shanks and cover the pot with a lid. Bake in the oven for 2 to 2½ hours, until the meat is very tender and falling off the bone.

5. Remove the shanks from the pot and set aside. Bring the braising liquid to a rolling boil over high heat. If using, whisk the arrowroot and water until smooth, then add to the braising liquid and cook, whisking, until it has thickened and can coat the back of a spoon. Season to taste.

6. **For the gremolata:** In a small bowl, combine the pomegranate seeds, parsley, lemon zest and juice, and garlic. Stir in the olive oil and season with the salt and pepper.

7. Plate the lamb shanks with the gremolata on top. Serve alongside your favorite grain or roasted vegetable.

Tip: *The shanks can be made up to 2 days ahead and refrigerated in an airtight container. Simply reheat to serve. The recipe can also be made in a slow cooker: Cook on low for 8 hours or high for 4 hours, checking often.*

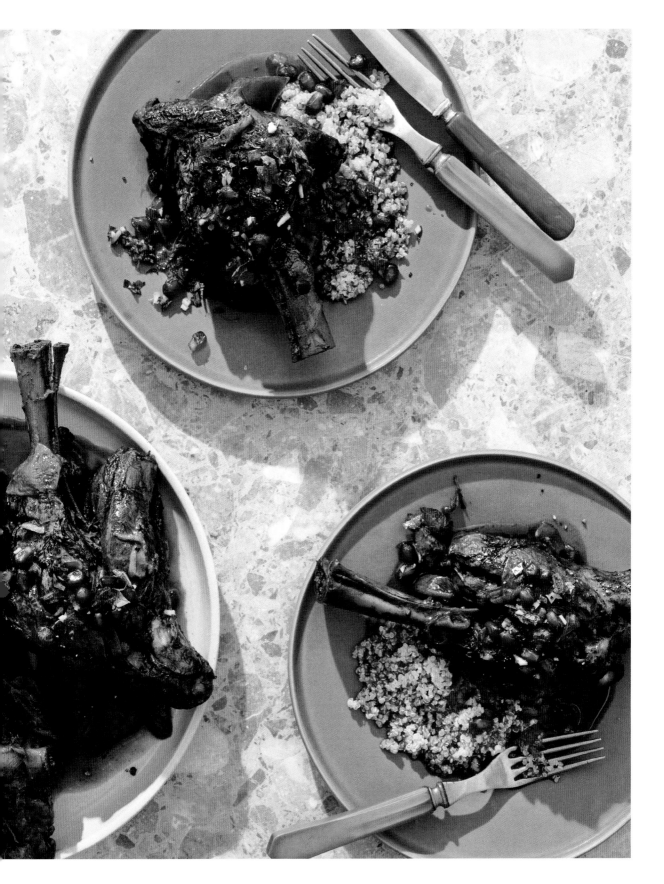

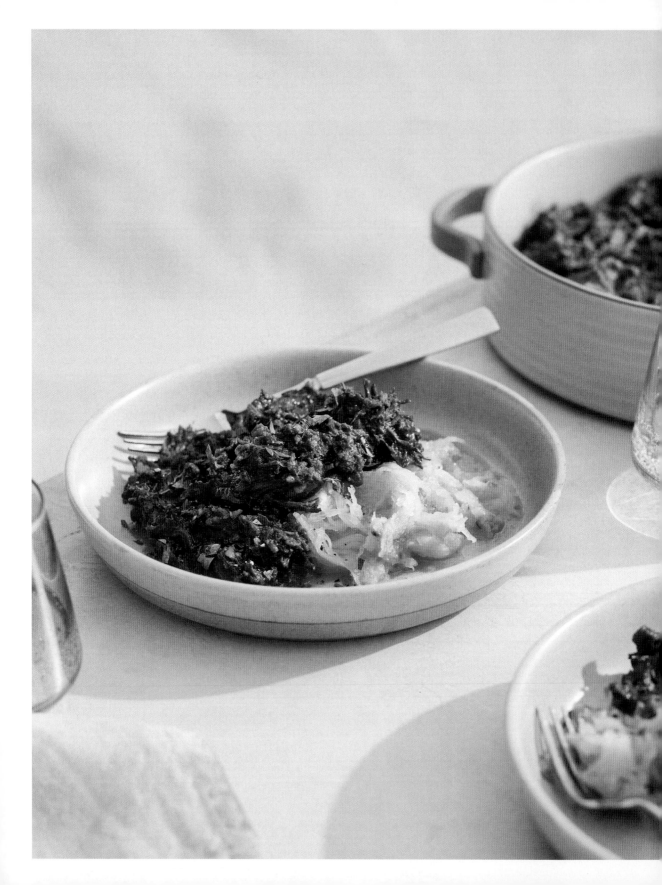

Beef Short Rib Ragu

Serves: 4 to 6

Prep Time: 25 minutes

Cook Time: 4 hours

Ragu

3 pounds grass-fed bone-in beef short rib, cut crosswise into 3-inch pieces

1½ teaspoons kosher salt

1 teaspoon freshly ground black pepper

1 tablespoon avocado oil

1 yellow onion, diced

1 small fennel bulb, cored and diced

¼ cup dry red wine

3 garlic cloves, minced

2 anchovy fillets, roughly chopped

1 (28-ounce) can *plus* 1 (14.5-ounce) can whole peeled Italian tomatoes, crushed by hand

1 medium carrot, peeled and roughly chopped

1 tablespoon tomato paste

2 sprigs fresh thyme

1 bay leaf

Spaghetti Squash

1 spaghetti squash, halved lengthwise

1 tablespoon extra-virgin olive oil

½ teaspoon kosher salt

In this ultimate comfort food, beef short ribs are slow-cooked with cubes of fennel and tomato until tender. It's a perfect dish for entertaining in the cooler months as it can be made well in advance. I like to serve this with nutritious spaghetti squash, a great low-carbohydrate alternative to pasta that is packed with fiber and beta-carotene; but you can easily serve it with your favorite gluten-free pasta.

1. Preheat the oven to 350°F.

2. **For the ragu:** Season the beef all over with 1 teaspoon of the salt and ½ teaspoon of the pepper. Heat the avocado oil in a large Dutch oven or other ovenproof pot over medium heat. Working in batches, sear the beef for 3 minutes per side, until golden brown. Set aside on a plate.

3. Remove all but 2 tablespoons of fat from the pot. Add the onion and fennel and cook for 4 minutes, until softened and translucent. Deglaze the pan with the red wine, scraping up all the brown bits from the pot with a wooden spoon. Add the garlic and anchovies and stir. Add the tomatoes, carrot, tomato paste, thyme, and bay leaf and stir in the remaining ½ teaspoon salt and ½ teaspoon pepper. Bring to a boil and return the beef to the pot. Reduce to a simmer, cover, and cook in the oven until the beef is tender and falling apart, 2½ to 3 hours, checking every hour or so and adding ½ to 1 cup of water as needed. Set the ragu aside while you bake the squash.

4. **For the spaghetti squash:** Increase the heat to 400°F. Line a baking sheet with parchment paper. Place the squash on the sheet cut side up. Drizzle with the olive oil and season with the salt. Roast for 35 to 45 minutes, until fork tender. Allow to cool slightly, then, using a fork, gently scrape the squash into "noodles."

5. Remove the bones from the beef and discard. Fish out and discard the bay leaf. Using forks, gently shred the meat, mixing it well with the sauce. Gently reheat the ragu over medium heat. Spoon on top of the squash noodles and serve.

Tip: *The ragu can be made up to 3 days in advance and stored in an airtight container in the fridge. It can also be frozen for up to 3 months.*

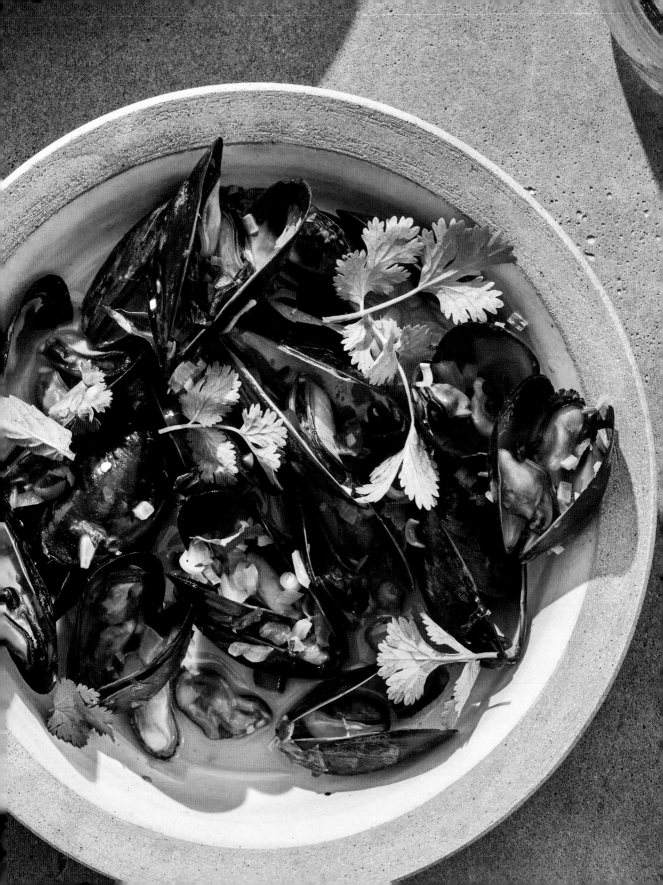

Seafood

Our whole-body health depends on a nutrient-dense diet, and certain types of seafood, like salmon, scallops, and mussels, can provide the essential omega-3 fatty acids, selenium, and vitamin D required for optimal cognitive performance and longevity. Sustainably raised and wild-caught varieties are safe, delicious, and nutritious options for a healthy diet. These recipes provide simple and fresh ways to create tasty meals for you and your family. Try my Steamed Fish with Ginger and Bok Choy (page 126) for a quick yet elegant main, or Tomato Fish Curry with Coconut Rice (page 131) for a warming one-pot meal. Fancy something for entertaining? Seared Scallops with Bursting Tomatoes (page 128) are a foolproof way to wow your friends. This section has something for everyone.

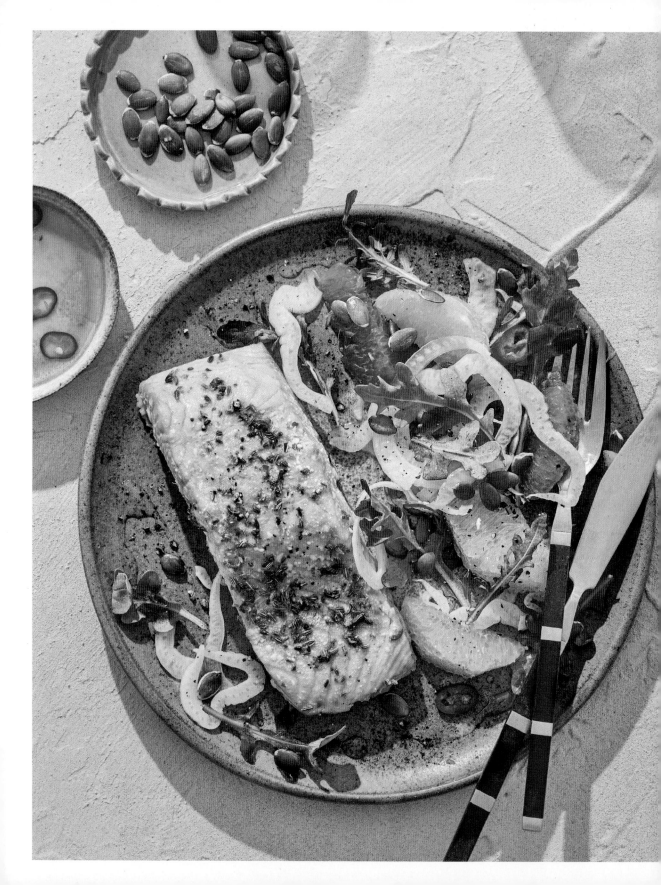

Salmon with Fennel and Citrus Salad

Serves: 4

Prep Time: 20 minutes

Cook Time: 20 minutes

Salmon

1 tablespoon extra-virgin olive oil

1 teaspoon ground fennel seed

1 teaspoon grated lime zest

½ teaspoon kosher salt

Pinch of freshly ground black pepper

Pinch of red pepper flakes

4 (6- to 8-ounce) fillets sustainably caught salmon

Dressing

3 tablespoons extra-virgin olive oil

2 tablespoons lime juice

1 teaspoon long red chile, seeded and thinly sliced (or ½ teaspoon red pepper flakes)

½ teaspoon kosher salt

½ teaspoon freshly ground black pepper

Salad

1 medium fennel bulb, cored and thinly shaved

2 cups baby arugula

⅓ cup fresh cilantro leaves

⅓ cup fresh mint leaves

1 grapefruit, peeled and segmented

1 orange, peeled and segmented

1 avocado, pitted, peeled, and sliced

¼ cup toasted pumpkin seeds

I love the simplicity of this dish, packed with bright citrus fruits and zesty herbs. Heart-healthy omega-3 fats from the salmon and avocado make it a substantial main course that will leave you feeling energized and satiated. Fennel and fennel seeds are loaded with potent plant compounds and antioxidants like vitamin C and manganese, which are vital for strong immune and bone health. Not only is raw fennel delicious and crunchy, but its versatile anise flavor makes it a stellar companion to salmon.

1. Preheat the oven to 350°F. Line a baking sheet with parchment paper.

2. **For the salmon:** In a small bowl combine the olive oil, fennel seed, lime zest, salt, black pepper, and pepper flakes. Gently spread the mixture over the salmon fillets and place the fillets on the baking sheet. Bake for 20 minutes, until the fish is flaky and reaches an internal temperature of 125°F.

3. **For the dressing:** Meanwhile, in a small bowl, whisk all the dressing ingredients together.

4. **For the salad:** In a large bowl, mix the fennel, arugula, cilantro, and mint. Add 2 tablespoons dressing and toss to coat. Transfer the fennel mixture to a large platter and top with the citrus segments. Add the avocado and sprinkle with the pumpkin seeds. Drizzle with the remaining dressing.

5. Divide the salad among four plates and top each with a salmon fillet.

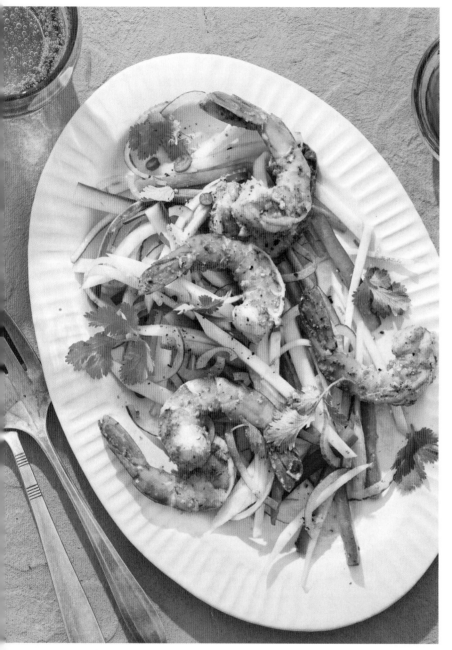

Serves: 4
Prep Time: 30 minutes
Cook Time: 5 minutes

Shrimp and Marinade

1 lemongrass stalk, outer layer removed, bulb and light green parts sliced

1 shallot, roughly chopped

⅓ cup fresh cilantro leaves

⅓ cup fresh mint leaves

3 garlic cloves, peeled

1 green chile, seeded and chopped

1 teaspoon grated fresh ginger

1 teaspoon ground cumin

1 teaspoon kosher salt

½ cup coconut cream

1 pound large wild-caught shrimp, shelled and deveined

The Young Forever Cookbook

Thai-Style Shrimp with Mango Salad

Mango Salad

2 large yellow mangoes, peeled, pitted, and thinly sliced

1 red bell pepper, stemmed, seeded, and thinly sliced

1 cup fresh cilantro leaves, plus more for garnish

1 small red onion, thinly sliced

¼ English cucumber, sliced into matchsticks

3 tablespoons extra-virgin olive oil

1 teaspoon grated lime zest

2 tablespoons lime juice

1 red Thai chile, seeded and thinly sliced

½ teaspoon kosher salt

¼ teaspoon freshly ground black pepper

1 tablespoon avocado oil

⅓ cup roughly chopped toasted cashews (optional)

This green-curry-style shrimp is easy to prepare and pairs perfectly with a sweet mango salad, bringing all the fresh flavors of Thailand right to your kitchen. Shrimp are a healthy, lean source of protein and a source of selenium and zinc, trace minerals that support the thyroid and a healthy immune system for life. I purchase wild-caught shrimp whenever possible, either fresh or frozen.

1. **For the shrimp:** In a food processor, combine the lemongrass, shallot, cilantro, mint, garlic, green chile, ginger, cumin, and salt. Pulse a few times, then add the coconut cream. Puree until a smooth paste forms, adding a splash of water if necessary.

2. Place the shrimp in a sealable bag, add the curry paste, and rub the mixture into the shrimp. Refrigerate for at least 15 minutes, while you make the salad, or up to 1 day.

3. **For the salad:** In a large bowl, mix the mangoes, bell pepper, cilantro, onion, and cucumber. Add the olive oil and lime zest and juice and toss to coat. Stir in the red chile to taste. Season with the salt and pepper.

4. Heat the avocado oil in a nonstick pan over medium heat. Add the shrimp with some of the marinade and cook for 2 to 3 minutes per side, until no longer opaque.

5. Divide the salad among bowls and top with the sautéed shrimp. Garnish with additional cilantro leaves and cashews, if desired.

Steamed Fish with Ginger and Bok Choy

Serves: 2 to 4

Prep Time: 10 minutes

Cook Time: 10 minutes

4 (5-ounce) fillets sustainably caught Mediterranean sea bass (branzino)

1 teaspoon kosher salt

4 heads bok choy, halved

¼ cup water

¼ cup gluten-free tamari

2 tablespoons mirin

1 teaspoon sesame oil

1 (2-inch) piece fresh ginger, peeled and julienned

1 bunch scallions, whites thinly sliced, greens julienned into 2-inch pieces

1 cup loosely packed fresh cilantro leaves with soft stems

2 tablespoons toasted sesame seeds

Chili oil, for serving

Cooked brown rice, for serving (optional)

Easy, healthy ways to cook fish are always a plus in my kitchen. Steamed fish takes only a few minutes and is delicious when topped with a piquant ginger scallion sauce. Finished with toasted sesame seeds, which are high in calcium and magnesium and contribute to healthy bones, this is a simple way to prepare fish at home. I like to use Mediterranean sea bass, also known as branzino, but you can easily substitute another mild, delicate white fish.

1. Season the sea bass fillets with the salt.

2. Fill a heavy bottomed pan with a lid with 1½ to 2 inches water. Bring to a boil, then reduce to a simmer. Add the bok choy, halved sides up. Cover and cook for 2 minutes. Place the fillets on top of the bok choy, cover, and steam until the fish is opaque, about 4 minutes.

3. In a small bowl, combine the water, tamari, and mirin. Heat the sesame oil in a pan over medium heat. Add the ginger and cook for 1 minute, until fragrant. Add the white parts of the scallions and continue cooking for 1 minute. Add the remaining julienned scallions, half of the cilantro, and the tamari mixture and cook until the scallion greens and cilantro are wilted, about 30 seconds.

4. Carefully remove the steamed fish from the pan and plate with some bok choy. Pour the sauce over the steamed fish. Sprinkle the remaining cilantro and toasted sesame seeds over the fish. Drizzle with chili oil and serve in bowls with brown rice if you like.

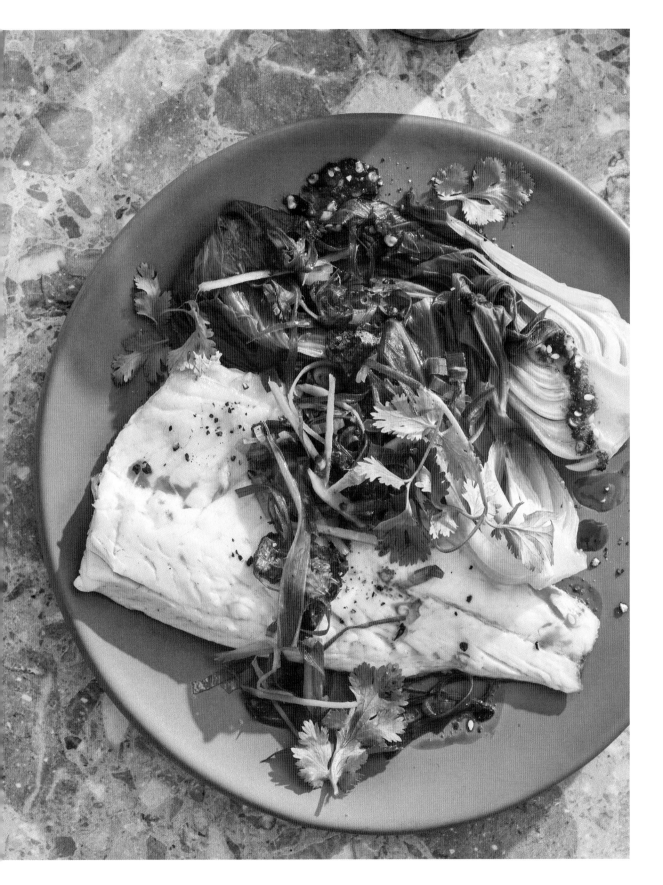

Seared Scallops with Bursting Tomatoes

Serves: 4

Prep Time: 10 minutes
Cook Time: 30 minutes

2 tablespoons extra-virgin olive oil

1 shallot, halved and thinly sliced

1 anchovy fillet

2 garlic cloves, thinly sliced

3 cups cherry tomatoes

½ cup kalamata olives, pitted and roughly chopped

2 tablespoons capers

½ teaspoon red pepper flakes

Kosher salt and freshly ground black pepper

12 large sea scallops, tough side muscles removed, patted dry

¼ cup finely chopped fresh flat-leaf parsley

1 lemon, cut into wedges

These Italian-inspired scallops are a simple main you can cook to impress, or simply enjoy on a weeknight. The bursting cherry tomatoes create a deliciously sweet sauce that pairs perfectly with naturally sweet scallops and briny olives. Scallops are a great source of lean protein, vitamin B_{12}, zinc, selenium, and anti-inflammatory omega-3 fatty acids, all of which contribute to a healthier immune system and improved cognitive health. This easy, yet beautiful main course is one you're going to want to add to your cooking repertoire.

1. Preheat the oven to 400°F.

2. Heat 1 tablespoon of the olive oil in a large cast-iron pan over medium heat. Add the shallot and sauté until translucent, about 3 minutes. Add the anchovy and garlic and continue to cook for another 2 minutes. Add the cherry tomatoes, olives, capers, and red pepper flakes and season with salt and pepper. Transfer the pan to the oven and bake for 15 minutes, until the tomatoes are beginning to split through the skins.

3. Season the scallops with salt and pepper. Heat the remaining 1 tablespoon olive oil in a nonstick pan over medium-high heat. Sear the scallops, cooking for 1 minute per side, until golden.

4. Remove the tomatoes from the oven and nestle the seared scallops into the tomatoes. Return the pan to the oven and bake for 3 to 4 minutes, until the scallops are opaque.

5. Sprinkle the scallops with the parsley and serve with lemon wedges.

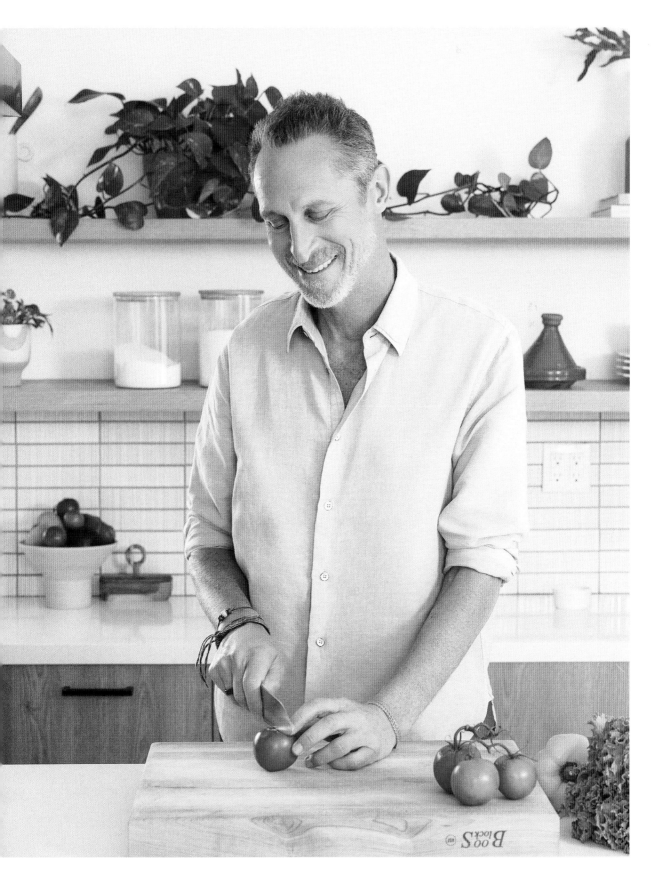

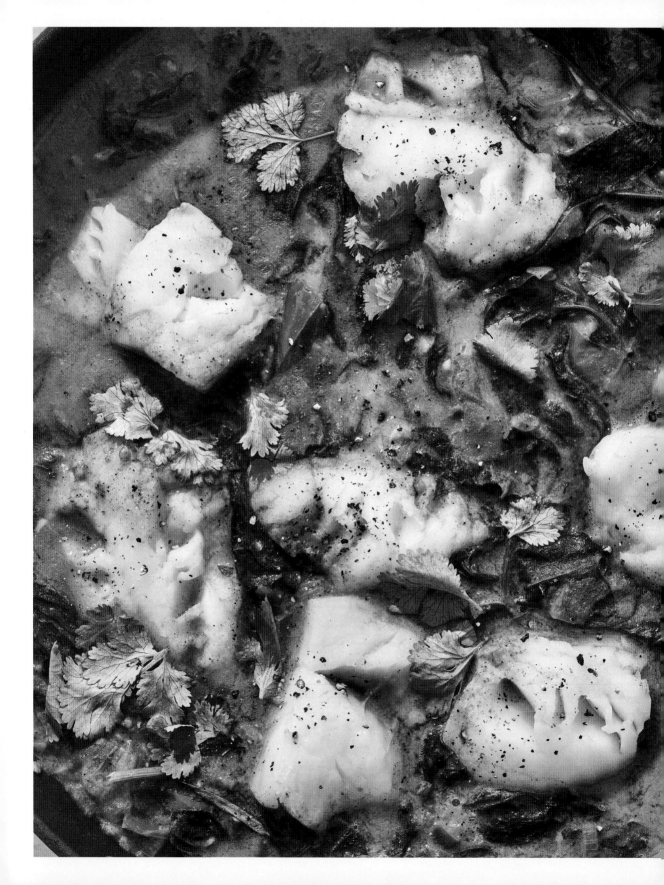

Tomato Fish Curry with Coconut Rice

Serves: 4

Prep Time: 15 minutes

Cook Time: 30 minutes

1½ cups brown basmati rice

1 (13.5-ounce) can full-fat unsweetened coconut milk

2½ cups water

1 tablespoon avocado oil

6 whole black peppercorns

2 whole cloves

1 cinnamon stick

1 yellow onion, finely chopped

1 garlic clove, minced

1 (1-inch) piece fresh ginger, peeled and finely chopped

1 tablespoon garam masala

1 teaspoon ground turmeric

1 teaspoon kosher salt

6 tomatoes, roughly chopped

½ teaspoon freshly ground black pepper

2 cups packed baby spinach

2 pounds skinless sustainably caught cod, salmon, or other firm fish, cut into 3-inch pieces

½ cup roughly chopped fresh cilantro leaves

1 lime, cut into wedges

This is one of my all-time favorite curries to cook at home. Comforting, healthy, and easy to prepare, it has become a mainstay in my household. Full of aromatic spices, fresh herbs, and creamy coconut, the flavorful but light South Indian curry makes the most delicious base for any firm fish, or shrimp or calamari. Common curry spices such as turmeric and ginger are full of antioxidants known for their anti-aging and anti-inflammatory benefits.

1. Combine the rice, ½ cup of the coconut milk, and the water in a pot, cover, and bring to a boil. Reduce the heat to a simmer and cook for 25 to 30 minutes, until all the liquid is absorbed.

2. Meanwhile, heat the avocado oil in a large pan with a tight-fitting lid over medium heat. Add the peppercorns, cloves, and cinnamon stick and cook for 1 minute, or until fragrant. Add the onion, garlic, and ginger and cook for 3 minutes, until the onion has softened. Reduce the heat to low and add the garam masala, turmeric, and salt. Stir for about 30 seconds, until lightly toasted.

3. Add the tomatoes to the pan and season with the pepper. Pour in the remaining coconut milk, cover, and simmer, stirring occasionally, for 15 to 20 minutes, until the tomatoes have broken down into a light sauce. Stir in the spinach to wilt slightly, then nestle the fish pieces into the sauce. Cover and cook for 6 to 8 minutes, until the fish flesh is firm.

4. To serve, scoop the coconut rice into bowls and top with the fish curry. Garnish with cilantro and lime wedges.

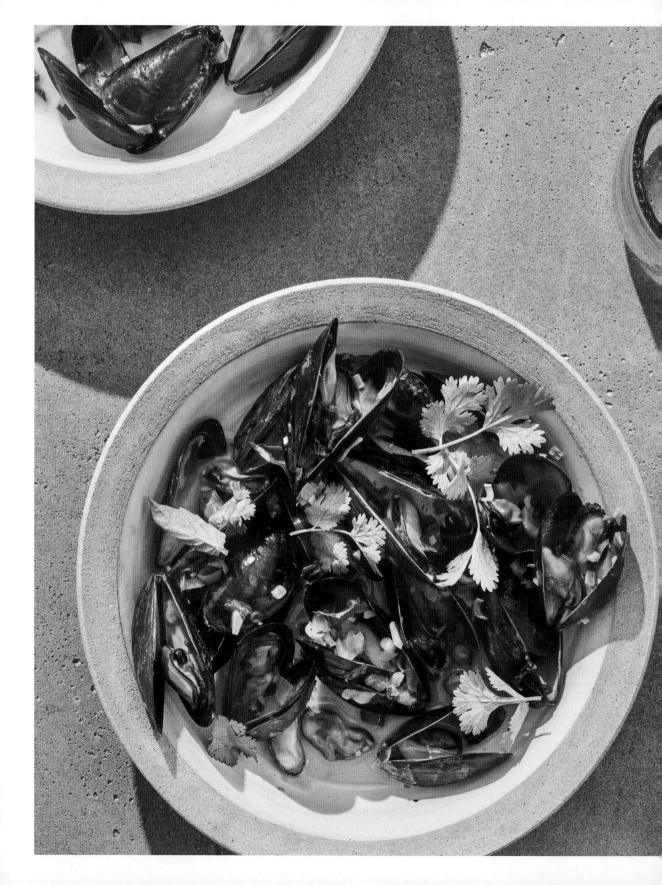

Mussels with Lemongrass and Ginger Broth

Serves: 4

Prep Time: 20 minutes

Cook Time: 10 minutes

2½ pounds mussels, debearded

1 tablespoon sesame oil

1 lemongrass stalk, outer layer removed, bulb and light green parts finely chopped

1 shallot, finely chopped

2 garlic cloves, thinly sliced

1 tablespoon finely chopped fresh ginger

1 tablespoon finely chopped fresh cilantro stems, leaves reserved

1 red Thai chile, seeded and thinly sliced

1½ cups full-fat unsweetened coconut milk

1 tablespoon gluten-free tamari

1 tablespoon lime juice

½ cup fresh Thai basil leaves

Mussels are impressively nutritious: high in protein, vitamin B$_{12}$, iron, and omega-3 fatty acids, to name a few. I've paired them with a light coconut broth infused with lemongrass, ginger, and chile. This dish comes together in no time and is a great way to include mussels in your cooking rotation.

1. Place the mussels in a colander, discarding any with open shells, and rinse a few times under cold running water to remove any sand or debris.

2. Heat the sesame oil in a large pot with a lid over medium heat. Add the lemongrass, shallot, garlic, ginger, cilantro stems, and chile. Cook until soft, about 3 minutes. Add the coconut milk and mussels, cover, and cook for 6 to 8 minutes, until the shells open. Discard any unopened shells.

3. Using a slotted spoon, spoon the mussels into wide, shallow bowls. Stir the tamari, lime juice, basil, and reserved cilantro leaves into the broth. Ladle the broth over the mussels and serve.

Tip: *The best way to store mussels is to remove them from the packaging and place them in a clean bowl. Cover with a damp paper towel and store at the back of your fridge. Use within one day. This dish is also delicious with clams if you prefer!*

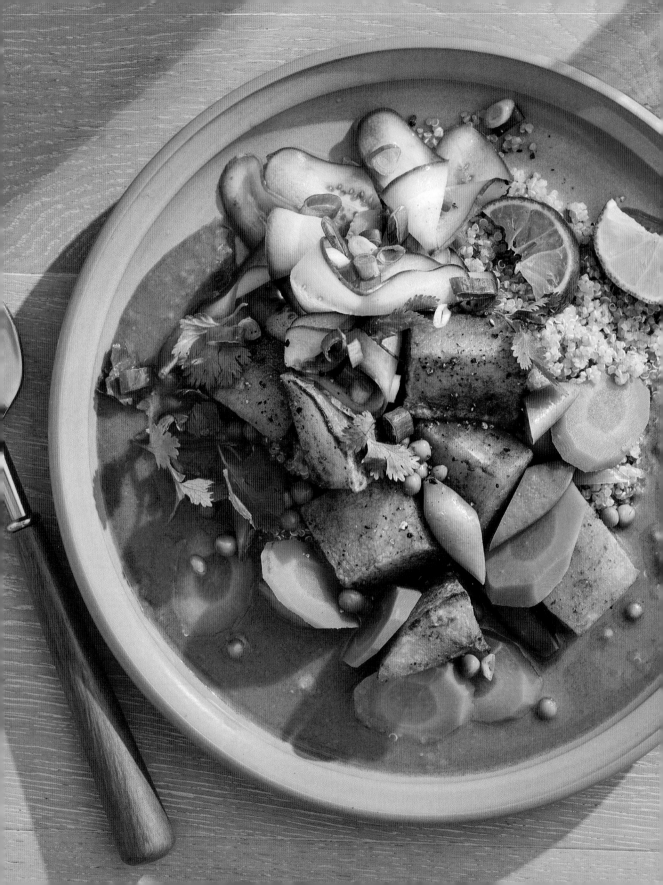

Vegetable Mains

One of the keys to longevity is maintaining a plant-rich diet. Consuming an array of colorful fruits and vegetables daily can provide plant-based protein, plenty of healthy fats, and all the beneficial phytonutrients and antioxidants necessary for an optimal health span. These vibrant veggie mains are packed with flavor and nutrients. My Mushroom Stroganoff (page 139) will convert any carnivore, while Stewed Black-Eyed Peas with Swiss Chard (page 141) provides a warm, nourishing meal. These diverse and hearty mains will keep your body happy for years to come.

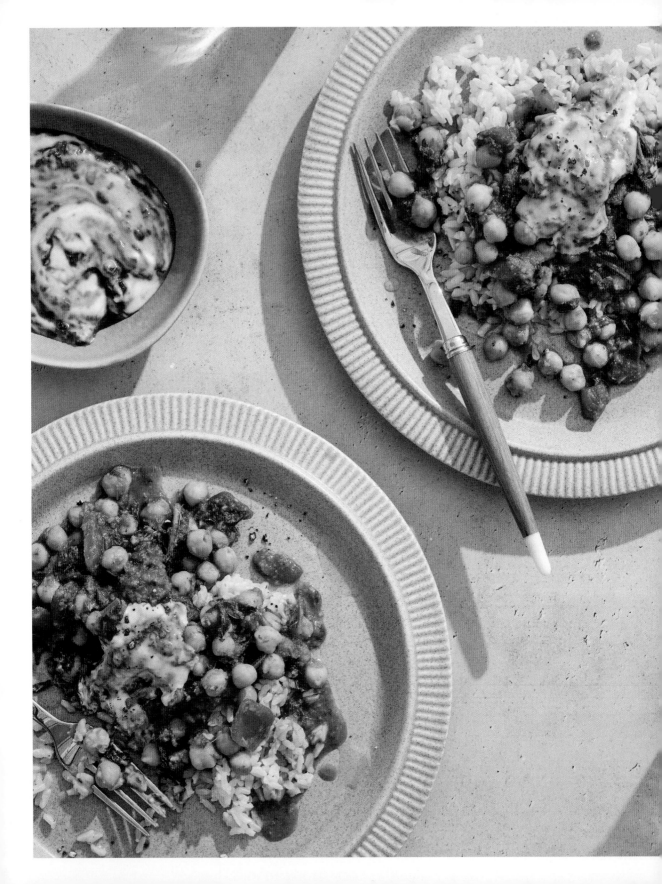

Chickpea Curry
with Beet Raita

Serves: 4
Prep Time: 15 minutes
Cook Time: 30 minutes

Chickpea Curry

2 shallots, roughly chopped

1 (1-inch) piece fresh ginger, peeled and roughly chopped

3 garlic cloves, chopped

1 green chile, seeded and roughly chopped

⅓ cup fresh cilantro leaves and soft stems

1 teaspoon ground coriander

1 teaspoon ground cumin

½ teaspoon kosher salt, plus more to taste

About 1 tablespoon water

10 fresh curry leaves

1 (14.5-ounce) can chopped tomatoes

1 (15.5-ounce) can chickpeas, drained and rinsed

1 cup vegetable stock

1 tablespoon garam masala

2 cups baby spinach, chopped

Beet Raita

¾ cup sheep's milk yogurt

1 tablespoon lime juice

½ teaspoon ground coriander

½ teaspoon kosher salt

½ cup peeled and thickly grated beets

This is my take on a chana masala, a hearty curry of chickpeas seasoned with garam masala. I've paired it with a cool beet raita, with the beets providing a vibrant pop of color and a natural sweetness that cuts the heat of the masala. The chickpeas in the curry provide plenty of fiber and protein, while the beets offer up antioxidants. The curry is filling enough on its own but pairs excellently with rice, quinoa, or keto flatbread.

1. **For the curry:** In a food processor, combine the shallots, ginger, garlic, green chile, and cilantro. Pulse a few times before adding the coriander, cumin, and salt. Blend until smooth, scraping down the sides occasionally and adding a tablespoon or two of water to turn it into a paste.

2. Heat a pan over medium heat. Add the paste and cook for 3 to 4 minutes, until softened and fragrant. Stir in the curry leaves and tomatoes and cook for 3 minutes, stirring often. Add the chickpeas and stock, bring to a boil, then reduce to a simmer. Cook, covered, for 15 minutes, until the mixture has thickened slightly and the chickpeas have softened. Stir in the garam masala and the spinach and cook until the spinach is wilted, about a minute. Season to taste with salt.

3. **For the raita:** In a bowl, stir together the yogurt, lime juice, coriander, and salt. Gently fold in the beets. Serve the curried chickpeas in bowls topped with raita.

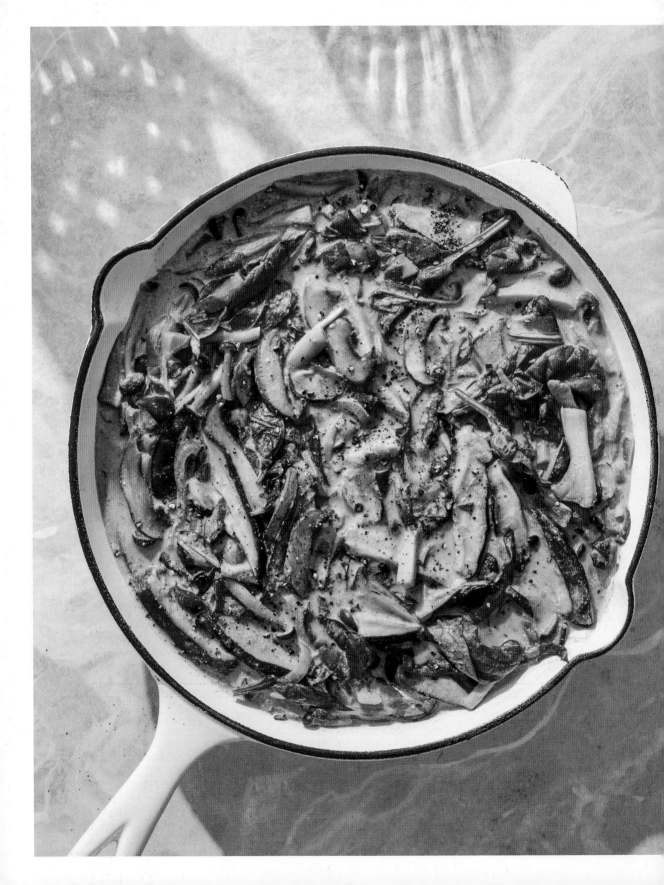

Mushroom Stroganoff

Serves: 4

Prep Time: 15 minutes
Cook Time: 30 minutes

1 (8-ounce) package organic soft tofu, drained

1 cup vegetable stock

1 cup brown basmati rice

2 cups water

1 tablespoon avocado oil

2 small yellow onions, thinly sliced

3 garlic cloves, roughly chopped

Kosher salt and freshly ground black pepper

1½ pounds mixed mushrooms (such as cremini, portobello, and oyster), roughly chopped

3 gherkins, finely chopped (optional)

1 teaspoon sweet paprika

Pinch of cayenne pepper

½ cup dry white wine

1½ teaspoons Dijon mustard

1 to 2 fresh thyme sprigs

1 heaping cup baby spinach, roughly chopped

2 tablespoons finely chopped fresh flat-leaf parsley

1 teaspoon grated lemon zest

1 teaspoon lemon juice, or to taste

⅓ cup roughly chopped toasted cashews, for serving

You won't be missing the beef in this unique twist on the classic stroganoff when hearty, tender mushrooms are simmered in a dairy-free, protein-packed sauce made with soft tofu. What I love about this dish is that the super creamy, flavorful sauce is nutrient-dense from the tofu and spinach. Perfect on a cool night, this warming stew can be served on its own or with brown rice, as suggested.

1. In a blender, puree the tofu and vegetable stock until smooth; set the puree aside.

2. Combine the rice and water in a saucepan and bring to a boil. Reduce to a simmer, cover, and cook for 25 to 30 minutes, until tender.

3. Meanwhile, heat the avocado oil in a large skillet over medium heat. Add the onions and cook until translucent and slightly golden, 6 to 8 minutes. Add the garlic and 1 teaspoon salt and cook for 1 minute, until fragrant. Transfer the onions to a bowl.

4. To the same pan, add the mushrooms and sauté for about 7 minutes, until golden brown. Reduce the heat slightly and stir in the garlic-onion mixture, along with the gherkins, if using, and the paprika and cayenne. Mix well and continue to cook for another 2 minutes. Deglaze the pan with the white wine and cook until most of the liquid has evaporated, about 2 minutes.

5. Stir in the mustard, then add the tofu puree and bring to a boil. Add the thyme, reduce to a simmer, and cook for 6 to 8 minutes, until the liquid is reduced and thickened slightly. Stir in the spinach and cook until wilted, about 1 minute. Add the parsley and lemon zest and juice. Season with salt and pepper, to taste.

6. Divide the rice among bowls, top with the mushroom stroganoff and a sprinkle of toasted cashews, and serve.

Chickpea Socca with Broccolini and Chermoula

Serves: 4

Prep Time: 30 minutes, including resting time

Cook Time: 15 minutes

Socca Batter

1 cup chickpea flour

1 cup water, plus more if needed

1½ tablespoons extra-virgin olive oil

¾ teaspoon kosher salt

Broccolini

1 bunch broccolini, thinly sliced lengthwise

1 tablespoon avocado oil

½ teaspoon kosher salt

Pinch of freshly ground black pepper

1 tablespoon avocado oil

½ cup Chermoula (page 206)

Fresh herbs, such as cilantro or flat-leaf parsley leaves

Lemon wedges

Socca is a gluten-free chickpea flatbread that is simple to make and so versatile. Chickpea flour can be found at most grocers now and is a great high-protein flour alternative. With a slightly nutty taste, socca pairs really well with roasted vegetables and a flavorful sauce, like my favorite chermoula. The batter for the socca can be made up to 2 hours ahead and left at room temperature. You can bake one large flatbread as directed, or try forming smaller individual breads.

1. **For the socca batter:** In a large mixing bowl, combine the flour, water, olive oil, and salt to create a thick pancake batter, adding more water if necessary. Allow to sit for 30 minutes.

2. **For the broccolini:** Meanwhile, in a bowl, toss the broccolini with the avocado oil and season with the salt and pepper. Spread the broccolini out on an unlined baking sheet in an even layer and set aside.

3. Preheat the oven to 400°F.

4. Add the avocado oil to an oven-safe frying pan (preferably cast iron). Heat over medium heat until almost smoking. Using a ladle, add the socca batter and gently swirl it until it reaches the edges.

5. Place both the socca pan and the broccolini sheet in the oven and bake until both are golden and crispy, 10 to 15 minutes. Roughly chop the broccolini and set aside.

6. Carefully transfer the socca to a platter. Add a good dollop of chermoula on top, spreading it almost to the edges. Top with the crispy broccolini, extra chermoula, and a sprinkle of fresh herbs. Serve with lemon wedges for squeezing.

Stewed Black-Eyed Peas with Swiss Chard

Serves: 4

Prep Time: 15 minutes

Cook Time: 30 minutes

Black-Eyed Peas

1 tablespoon extra-virgin olive oil

1 large leek, white and light green parts only, halved lengthwise and thinly sliced

1 celery stalk, halved lengthwise and finely chopped

2 garlic cloves, minced

2 to 3 teaspoons seeded and finely chopped red chile

1 bunch Swiss chard, leaves roughly chopped, stems finely chopped

1 cup strained tomatoes

2 (15.5-ounce) cans black-eyed peas, drained and rinsed

2 cups vegetable stock

Gremolata

½ cup finely chopped fresh flat-leaf parsley

2 garlic cloves, minced

2 teaspoons grated lemon zest

2 teaspoons lemon juice

Beans and greens are a classic combination, and this one doesn't disappoint. Beans like black-eyed peas are highly nutritious legumes containing high amounts of fiber that can reduce inflammation and are good for your gut microbiome. Simmered canned beans cooked with soft leeks and a hint of chile heat means this dish comes together quickly. Any sturdy green will work here; Tuscan kale and dandelion are good substitutions for the Swiss chard, but omit the stalks if cooking these. With a bracing garnish of fresh parsley, garlic, and lemon that brightens the dish, these stewed black-eyed peas are anything but boring.

1. **For the black-eyed peas:** Heat the olive oil in a large pan with a lid over medium heat. Add the leek and celery and cook until softened, about 4 minutes. Add the garlic and chile and cook for 1 minute, then add 1 cup of the finely chopped chard stems, saving the rest for your next stir-fry or soup. Stir and cook for 4 minutes, until the stems are tender. Add the chard leaves, stir, and cook for 2 minutes, until they begin to wilt. Add the strained tomatoes and stir to coat.

2. Add the black-eyed peas and stock and stir well until combined. Bring to a boil, then reduce to a simmer and cook, covered, for 15 minutes. Remove the lid and continue cooking for 5 minutes, until slightly thickened.

3. **For the gremolata:** In a small bowl, stir all the ingredients together.

4. Serve the stewed peas in bowls topped with the gremolata. If you're feeling extra hungry, add a scoop of cooked quinoa or brown rice.

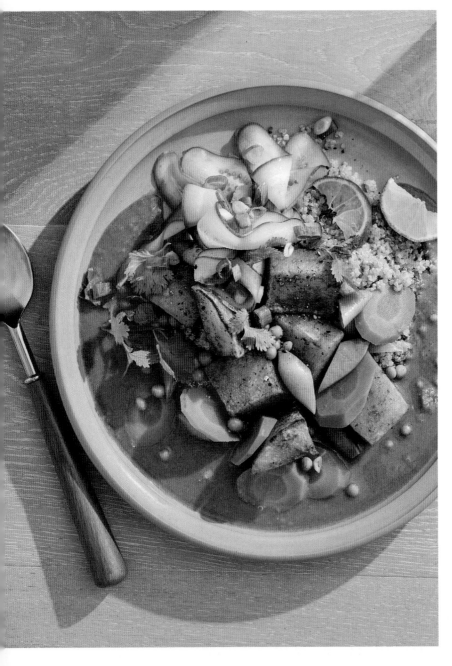

Serves: 4 to 6

Prep Time: 25 minutes

Cook Time: 30 minutes

Squash

1 (2½-pound) butternut squash, peeled and cut into 1½-inch cubes

2 tablespoons avocado oil

1 teaspoon turmeric

½ teaspoon cayenne

½ teaspoon ground coriander

1 teaspoon kosher salt

½ teaspoon freshly ground black pepper

Curry

1 (13.5-ounce) can full-fat unsweetened coconut milk, chilled at least 3 hours

½ cup vegetable stock

1 cup cannellini beans, drained and rinsed

5 tablespoons Thai yellow curry paste

1 teaspoon maple syrup (optional)

2 teaspoons gluten-free tamari

1 large carrot, peeled and thinly sliced on the bias

1 cup snap peas, ends trimmed

¾ cup frozen peas

Butternut Squash Curry with Cucumber Relish

Cucumber Relish

3 mini cucumbers, shaved into ribbons

5 scallions, white and light green parts, thinly sliced on the bias

½ cup fresh cilantro leaves

2 tablespoons rice wine vinegar

To Serve

Brown rice or quinoa (optional)

½ cup roughly chopped toasted cashews

1 lime, cut into wedges

This curry has all the flavors of Thailand packed into one dish. To make things easy, I've used a good-quality store-bought curry paste and amped up the flavor with spiced squash. I've even hidden some extra protein in the coconut sauce with pureed white beans, making this an incredibly nutritious curry. Topped with a quick, fresh cucumber salad, it's an ideal weeknight meal that's also great as leftovers.

1. **For the squash:** Preheat the oven to 425°F and place a rack on the lower third of the oven. Line a baking sheet with parchment paper.

2. In a large bowl, toss the squash with the avocado oil, then add the spices and salt and pepper. Mix well so all the squash pieces are evenly coated. Transfer to the lined baking sheet and roast for 25 to 30 minutes, turning halfway, until tender.

3. **For the curry:** Scoop out the firm coconut cream from the top of the can and place in a bowl. Pour the remaining liquid from the can into a blender and add the vegetable stock and beans. Puree until very smooth.

4. Heat a large pan over medium heat. Add the curry paste and cook for 2 to 3 minutes, until fragrant. Add the coconut cream and stir until it has melted completely. Pour in the bean puree and bring to a boil. Add the maple syrup, if using, and the tamari, stirring well. Bring to a boil, reduce to a simmer, and add the carrot. Cook for 1 minute then add the snap peas and cook for 4 minutes, until the snap peas are slightly tender. Stir in the frozen peas and cook for 2 minutes, until completely defrosted.

5. **For the cucumber relish:** Arrange the cucumber and scallions in a bowl lined with a paper towel and let sit for 5 minutes to absorb extra moisture. Remove the paper towel, then gently mix in the cilantro and vinegar.

6. **To serve:** If using a grain, add a scoop to bowls. Top each with a ladleful of curry, a few pieces of roasted squash, and a spoonful of cucumber relish. Sprinkle with toasted cashews and serve with lime wedges.

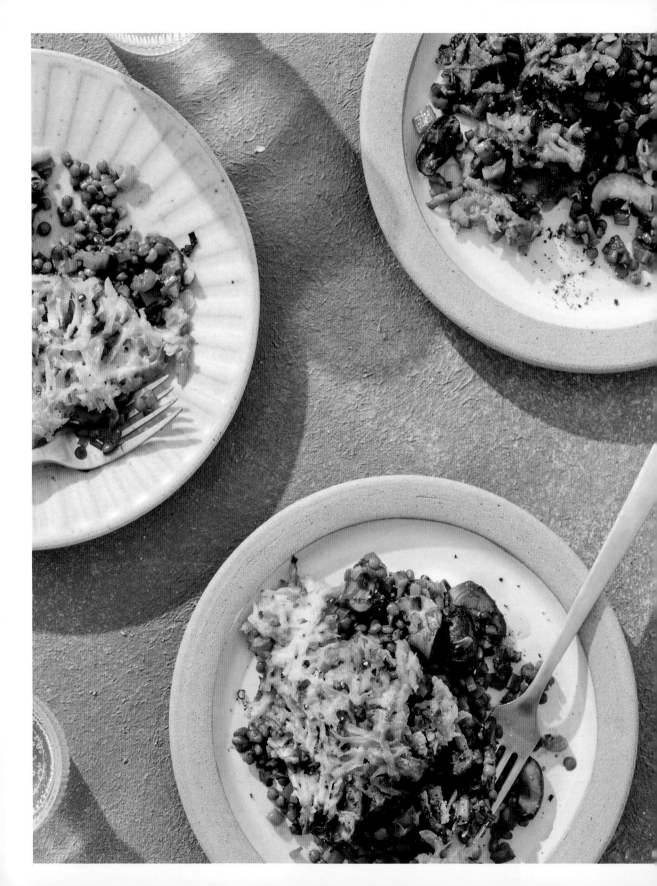

Mushroom, Lentil, and Parsnip Rosti

The flavors of French cooking come through in this one-pan mushroom and lentil stew with a crispy, crunchy parsnip topping. Sweet parsnips sub in for the traditional white potatoes and protein-rich lentils and mushrooms are the base, which is reminiscent of beef bourguignon—except with meaty mushrooms. Mushrooms are a superfood containing three different sources of B vitamins and vitamin D, which help the body better absorb calcium, leading to healthier bones for life. Packed with extra protein from canned lentils, this is a great weeknight meal suitable for all family members.

Serves: 4

Prep Time: 25 minutes

Cook Time: 1 hour

3 tablespoons extra-virgin olive oil

1¼ pounds cremini mushrooms, sliced

Kosher salt and freshly ground black pepper

1 carrot, peeled and finely chopped

1 large leek, finely chopped

1 celery stalk, finely chopped

1 garlic clove, minced

1 teaspoon fresh thyme leaves

1 tablespoon tomato paste

1 tablespoon whole-grain mustard

½ cup dry red wine

1 (15.5-ounce) can brown lentils, drained and rinsed

2 cups vegetable stock

1 large pasture-raised organic egg

1 tablespoon arrowroot powder

3 large parsnips, peeled and grated

1. Preheat the oven to 400°F.

2. Heat 1 tablespoon of the olive oil in a 12-inch cast-iron pan over medium heat. Add the mushrooms and cook, stirring, for 8 minutes, until soft and golden at the edges. Season with 1 teaspoon salt and ½ teaspoon pepper. Remove the mushrooms from the pan and set aside.

3. In the same pan, heat 1 tablespoon of the olive oil over medium heat. Add the carrot, leek, and celery and sauté until soft, 4 to 6 minutes. Stir in the garlic and thyme.

4. Return the mushrooms to the pan, stir in, then add the tomato paste and mustard. Increase the heat slightly and deglaze the pan with the wine, scraping up any bits that stick to the bottom. Boil until most of the liquid has evaporated, about 2 minutes.

5. Stir in the lentils, then add the stock and season with ½ teaspoon salt and ½ teaspoon pepper. Bring to a boil and cook for 2 minutes then remove from the heat.

6. In a small bowl, whisk the egg with the arrowroot powder. In a large bowl, combine the parsnips with ½ teaspoon salt and the remaining 1 tablespoon olive oil. Stir in the egg and arrowroot mixture.

7. Scatter the parsnips all over the mushrooms, leaving a ½-inch border around the edge. Cover the pan with foil and bake for 15 minutes. Remove the foil and continue baking for 15 to 20 minutes, until the top is golden brown. Serve immediately.

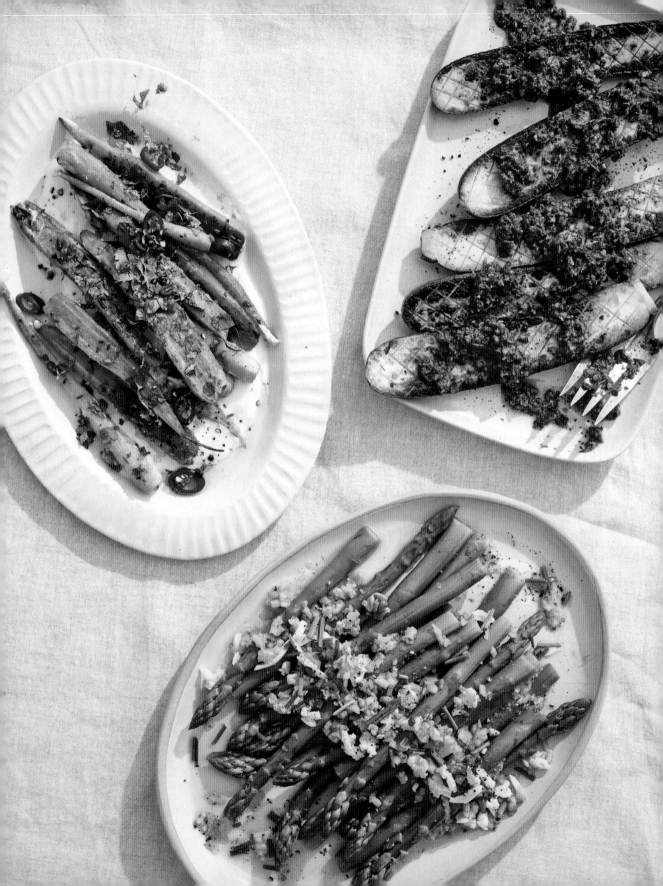

Sides

A colorful, nutrient-dense side dish can really make a meal. Whether you're looking for something to complement grilled fish, roasted chicken, or a hearty vegetable main, there is something here for you. These recipes don't shy away from flavor and are all vegetable-forward. My goal in this chapter is to showcase the versatility and adaptability of vegetables to different cooking techniques and flavors. We've got Roasted Cabbage Wedges with Tempeh "Bacon" (page 159), an indulgent Cauliflower Gratin (page 157), and Asparagus Vinaigrette (page 163), a twist on a classic French dish.

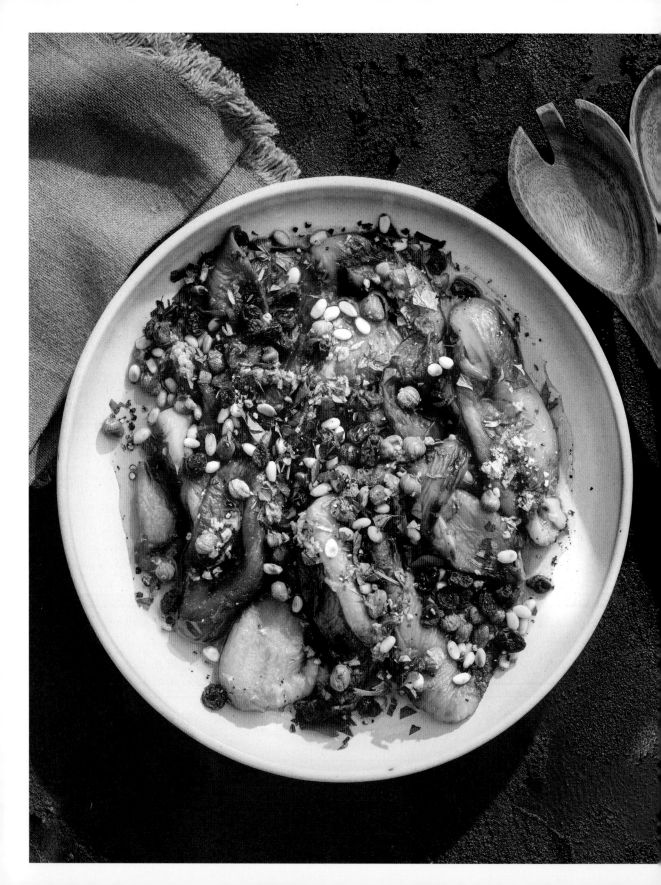

Roasted Pepper Medley
with Pine Nut Salsa

Serves: 4

Prep Time: 15 minutes

Cook Time: 45 minutes

6 red, yellow, or orange
bell peppers

3 tablespoons extra-virgin
olive oil

3 anchovy fillets, finely chopped

1 tablespoon capers

1 tablespoon sherry vinegar

1 teaspoon grated lemon zest

1 teaspoon lemon juice

½ teaspoon kosher salt

¼ teaspoon freshly ground
black pepper

¼ cup toasted pine nuts

¼ cup raisins, soaked in warm
water and drained

3 tablespoons finely chopped
fresh flat-leaf parsley

Bell peppers are rich in vitamin C and packed with antioxidants like carotenoids, which can help with your cardiovascular health, making them an
excellent snack or addition to any meal. Grilling them over a flame or
roasting them in the oven helps concentrate their flavor, leaving them
sweet and silky, perfect for mopping up the delicious southern Italian
inspired anchovy vinaigrette.

1. Preheat the grill to high or oven to 450°F.

2. Coat the peppers with 1 tablespoon of the olive oil. Grill until the skins
are blackened, about 35 minutes, rotating the peppers every 10 minutes
or so. Or to roast the peppers in the oven: Place the whole peppers on a
baking sheet lined with foil and roast for 25 minutes, turning halfway, or
until the skins are charred and the peppers are soft.

3. Place the charred peppers in a large bowl. Cover with plastic wrap and
let steam until the peppers are cool enough to handle, about 10 minutes.
This will help you remove the skins more easily. Break each pepper open
and remove and discard the stems. Gently peel the blackened skin from
the peppers and wipe away any seeds. Place the peppers on a large platter
and let sit for up to 10 minutes; they will release quite a bit of liquid as
they rest.

4. Meanwhile, whisk the anchovies, capers, vinegar, lemon zest and
juice, and remaining 2 tablespoons oil together. Season with the salt and
pepper.

5. Gently blot the peppers dry, dry the platter, and return the peppers.
Pour the dressing all over the peppers. Scatter the pine nuts, raisins, and
parsley all over and serve at room temperature.

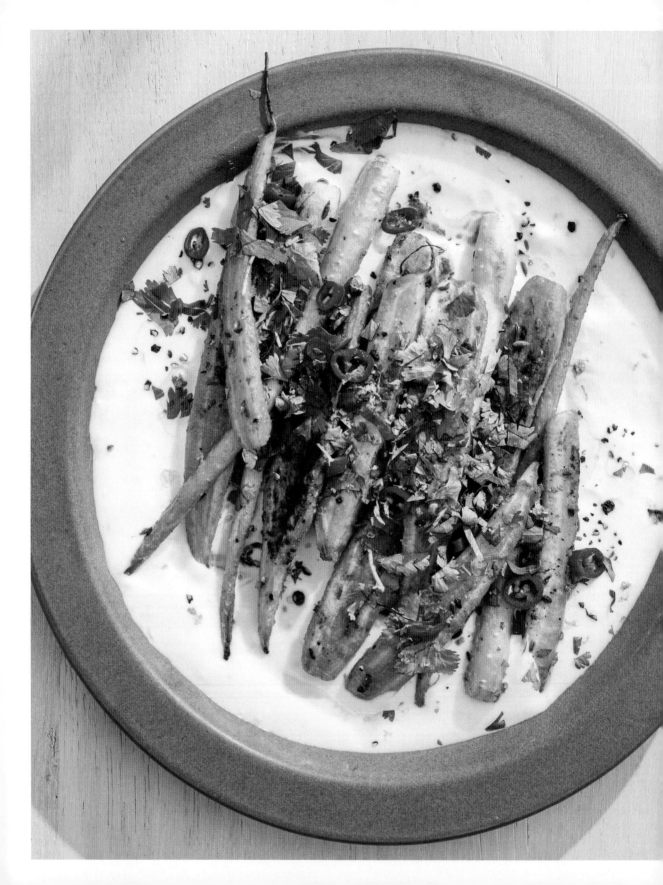

Caramelized Carrots with Lime Yogurt

Serves: 4

Prep Time: 15 minutes

Cook Time: 30 minutes

Carrots

2 tablespoons extra-virgin olive oil, plus more for serving

2 garlic cloves, grated

2 teaspoons ground cumin

1 teaspoon toasted cumin seeds

½ teaspoon fennel seeds

1 teaspoon grated lemon zest

2 teaspoons kosher salt

1½ pounds medium carrots, halved lengthwise if thick

Yogurt

1 cup sheep's milk yogurt

1 tablespoon lime juice

Pinch of red pepper flakes

Fresh cilantro leaves, for serving

In this easy-to-assemble side dish, caramelized carrots take center stage. Gently spiced with fennel and cumin, roasted carrots are both nutritious and delicious. Carrots are an excellent source of vitamin A and beta-carotene, which help promote healthy eyesight and regenerate damaged collagen, a protein essential to the skin's elasticity.

1. Preheat the oven to 425°F. Line a baking sheet with parchment paper.

2. **For the carrots:** In a large bowl, whisk together the olive oil, garlic, 1 teaspoon of the ground cumin, the cumin seeds, fennel seeds, lemon zest, and salt. Add the carrots and toss to evenly coat. Place the carrots, cut side down if sliced, on a rimmed baking sheet. Roast, flipping about halfway through, until the carrots are caramelized and tender, 25 to 30 minutes. Allow to cool slightly.

3. **For the yogurt:** In a small bowl, combine the yogurt, remaining 1 teaspoon ground cumin, the lime juice, and red pepper flakes to taste.

4. Spread the yogurt on the bottom of a rimmed plate. Top with roasted carrots and garnish with cilantro and a good drizzle of olive oil.

Brussels Sprouts with Pecorino and Hazelnuts

Serves: 4

Prep Time: 15 minutes

Cook Time: 15 minutes

1 pound Brussels sprouts, outer leaves removed and reserved, sprouts halved and thinly sliced

3 tablespoons extra-virgin olive oil

1 teaspoon kosher salt

¼ teaspoon freshly ground black pepper

2 tablespoons lemon juice

1 tablespoon Dijon mustard

1 teaspoon honey

1 garlic clove, minced

2 ounces pecorino or hard sheep's milk cheese, shaved

⅓ cup roughly chopped toasted hazelnuts

Brussels sprouts are packed with nutrients like gut-friendly fiber and immune-boosting vitamin C. Low in carbohydrates, they are a great addition to your weekly cruciferous veggie intake because they can be served both raw or cooked and are extremely versatile. I opt for both raw *and* cooked here, because I love the contrasting textures. Paired with creamy pecorino, a sheep's milk cheese from Italy, and toasted hazelnuts, another heart-healthy ingredient, this is a delicious side for grilled fish or meat.

1. Preheat the oven to 400°F. Line a baking sheet with parchment paper.

2. In a large bowl, combine the sprout leaves, 1 tablespoon of the olive oil, ½ teaspoon of the salt, and the pepper and toss to coat. Transfer to the baking sheet and roast, stirring often, for 15 minutes, or until crisp.

3. In the same bowl, combine the lemon juice, mustard, honey, garlic, and remaining 2 tablespoons olive oil. Season with the remaining ½ teaspoon salt and whisk until smooth. Add the sliced raw Brussels sprouts and mix well. Add the roasted sprout leaves and mix. Top with shavings of pecorino and hazelnuts and serve.

Roasted Purple Sweet Potatoes with Dukkah and Tahini

Serves: 4 to 6

Prep Time: 15 minutes

Cook Time: 35 minutes

2½ pounds purple sweet potatoes, halved and cut into wedges

2 tablespoons avocado oil

1 teaspoon kosher salt, plus more to taste

½ teaspoon ground black pepper, plus more to taste

⅓ cup tahini

2 tablespoons maple syrup

1 tablespoon apple cider vinegar

Up to ¼ cup water

¼ cup Almond Dukkah (page 209) or store-bought dukkah

1 cup roughly chopped fresh cilantro leaves

Sweet potatoes are one of my favorite root vegetables, and purple ones are both impressive in color and nutrition. They're a rich source of anti-oxidants and the vitamin A precursor beta carotene, which is essential for long-term immune health and good eyesight. Their purple flesh signals the presence of anthocyanins, which have been found to delay aging. The purple variety contains more starch, making them great for roasting.

1.   Preheat the oven to 425°F and arrange the racks on the bottom and top third of the oven. Line two baking sheets with parchment paper.

2.   In a large bowl, combine the potato wedges, avocado oil, ½ teaspoon of the salt, and the pepper and toss to coat. Transfer to the baking sheets and roast for 30 to 35 minutes, flipping the sheets halfway and rotating the wedges, until fork tender.

3.   Whisk the tahini, maple syrup, vinegar, and remaining ½ teaspoon salt in a small bowl. Gradually add the water until desired consistency is reached. Season with more salt and pepper if needed.

4.   To serve, arrange the potato wedges on a large platter. Drizzle with some of the tahini sauce, and sprinkle with almond dukkah and cilantro leaves.

Spiced Kohlrabi with Pomegranate and Feta

Serves: 4

Prep Time: 15 minutes

Cook Time: 30 minutes

2 tablespoons avocado oil

4 garlic cloves, smashed and roughly chopped

1 teaspoon fennel seeds

1 teaspoon cumin seeds

1 teaspoon black or brown mustard seeds

1 teaspoon ground turmeric

½ teaspoon kosher salt

2 pounds kohlrabi, peeled and cut into 1½-inch cubes

1 teaspoon grated lemon zest

1 tablespoon lemon juice

3 ounces sheep's or goat milk feta cheese

⅓ cup pomegranate seeds

Fresh mint leaves, for garnish

Fresh cilantro leaves, for garnish

Kohlrabi is perhaps not the most common vegetable, but it's one you should keep on your radar. A member of the cabbage family, kohlrabi shares similarities in texture and taste with turnips. It can be roasted or eaten raw and contains an abundance of nutrients: fiber, vitamins C and B$_6$ (which support immune health), and potassium (which is important for heart health). This is a delicious side dish with Middle Eastern spices, creamy feta, crunchy pomegranate seeds, and a topping of fresh herbs. It pairs well with marinated chicken, beef, or lamb.

1. Preheat the oven to 425°F. Line a baking sheet with parchment paper.

2. In a large bowl, whisk the avocado oil, garlic, fennel seeds, cumin seeds, mustard seeds, turmeric, and salt. Add the kohlrabi and toss to coat. Transfer to the baking sheet and roast for 30 minutes, stirring halfway, until fork tender.

3. Stir the lemon zest and juice into the kohlrabi on the baking sheet before transferring to a large serving bowl. Top with the feta, pomegranate seeds, mint, and cilantro and serve.

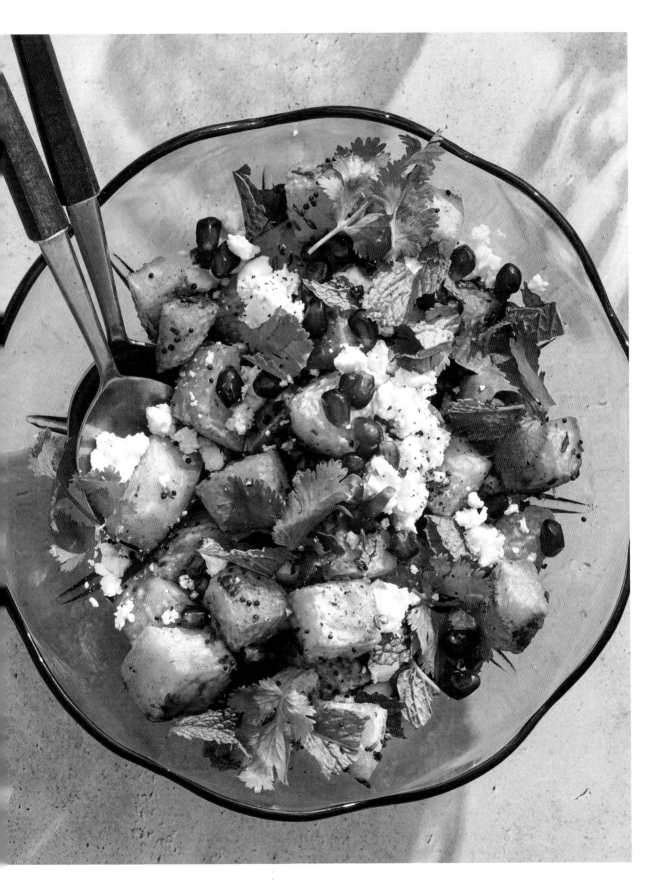

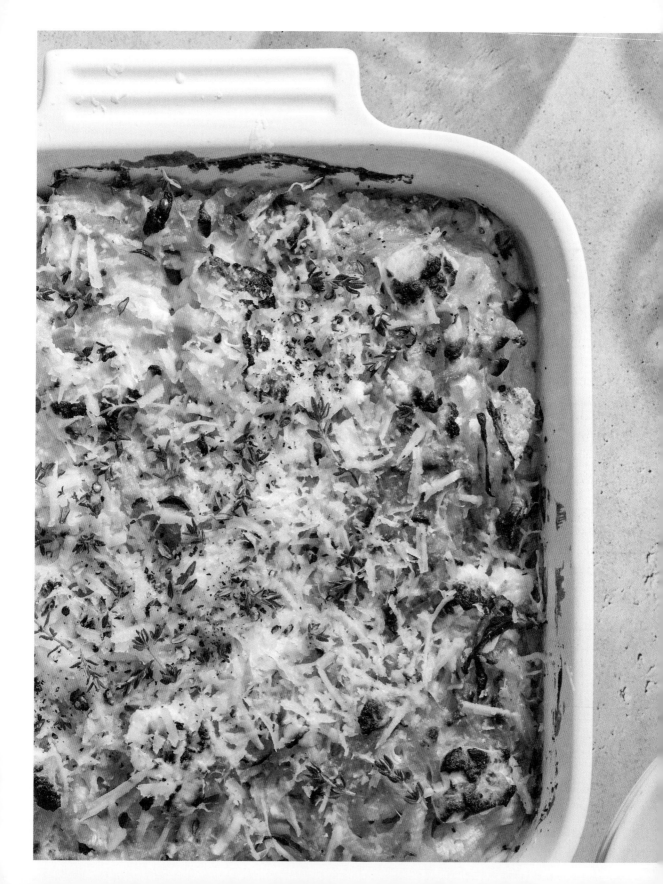

Cauliflower Gratin

Serves: 6

Prep Time: 15 minutes

Cook Time: 1 hour

2 tablespoons extra-virgin olive oil

1 head cauliflower, cut into medium florets

1 tablespoon grass-fed butter

2 onions, halved and thinly sliced

1 fennel bulb, cored and thinly sliced

4 garlic cloves, minced

2 cups unsweetened nondairy milk

¼ cup arrowroot powder

2 tablespoons Dijon mustard

1 teaspoon kosher salt

1 teaspoon freshly ground black pepper

3½ ounces goat cheese

¼ cup grated pecorino cheese

Leaves from 4 sprigs fresh thyme

This gratin is my better-for-you version of the typically decadent side dish, usually made with potatoes and cream. It feels elegant enough for a dinner party but is easy enough for a simple weeknight meal. If you want to keep it dairy-free, omit the cheeses and butter or use nondairy versions.

1. Preheat the oven to 400°F. In a 12-inch ovenproof baking dish, drizzle 1 tablespoon of olive oil to coat the bottom. Add the cauliflower to the baking dish and set aside.

2. Heat the remaining 1 tablespoon oil and the butter in a large pan over medium heat. Add the onions and fennel and cook until soft and golden, about 15 minutes. Add the garlic and cook for 1 minute, until fragrant. Remove the pan from the heat and let cool slightly.

3. Bring the milk to a boil in a pan over medium heat. Reduce to a simmer and whisk in the arrowroot powder. Whisk in the mustard and cook, whisking, for 2 minutes. Add the salt, pepper, and half the goat cheese and stir. Add the onion and fennel mixture and stir well.

4. Spread the onion mixture over the cauliflower with a spatula. Dot the remaining goat cheese on top. Cover the dish with foil and bake for 20 minutes. Remove the foil and sprinkle with the pecorino and thyme. Return to the oven and bake, uncovered, for 20 minutes, until golden brown and bubbling.

5. Allow to cool for at least 10 minutes before serving.

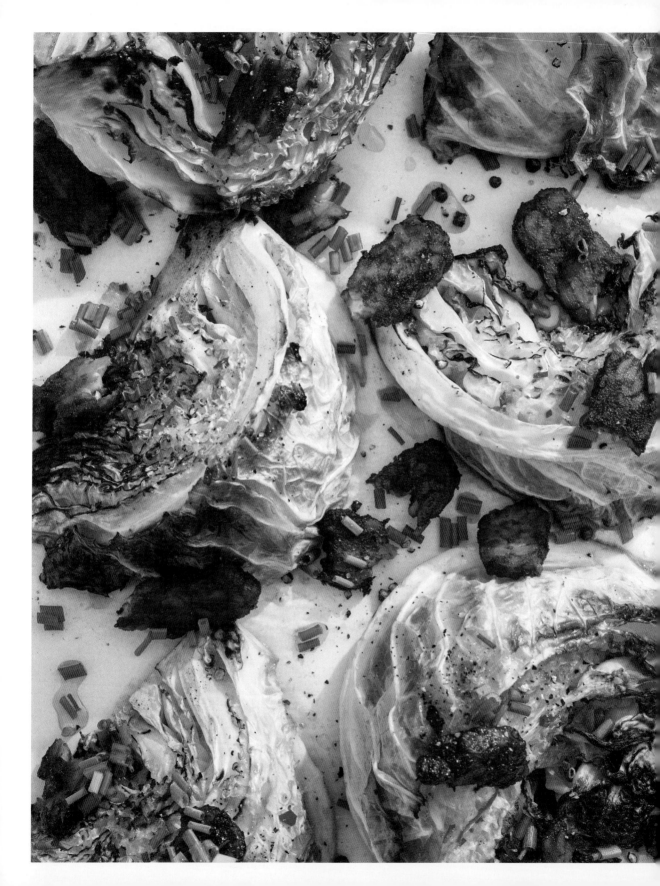

Roasted Cabbage Wedges with Tempeh "Bacon"

Serves: 6

Prep Time: 10 minutes

Cook Time: 55 minutes

Tempeh Bacon

3 tablespoons coconut aminos

2 tablespoons avocado oil

1 tablespoon apple cider vinegar

1 tablespoon maple syrup

2 teaspoons smoked paprika

1 teaspoon garlic powder

Pinch of cayenne

8 ounces tempeh, cut into
¼-inch-thick strips

Cabbage

1 to 2 tablespoons avocado oil

1 large green or savoy cabbage,
outer leaves removed, cut into
8 wedges

1 teaspoon grated lemon zest

¼ cup lemon juice

2 tablespoons extra-virgin
olive oil

4 garlic cloves, smashed and
roughly chopped

1 teaspoon kosher salt

½ teaspoon freshly ground
black pepper

Pinch of red pepper flakes

2 tablespoons finely chopped
fresh chives, for garnish

Roasting cabbage transforms the otherwise humble vegetable into something truly delicious. In this twist on the iceberg lettuce wedge salad, large wedges of cabbage are roasted with a lemony garlic dressing until crispy and golden, then paired with crunchy tempeh bacon. The cabbage is loaded with sweet, nutty flavors and contains gut-friendly fiber to aid in digestion and promote a healthy gut microbiome.

1. Preheat the oven to 400°F and arrange the oven racks in the middle and bottom of the oven. Line two baking sheets with parchment paper.

2. **For the tempeh bacon:** In a large shallow bowl or dish, whisk the coconut aminos, avocado oil, vinegar, maple syrup, paprika, garlic powder, and cayenne. Add the tempeh strips and gently toss to coat. Let marinate while you prepare the cabbage.

3. **For the cabbage:** In a large cast-iron pan, heat 1 tablespoon avocado oil. Working in batches, add the cabbage wedges and sear for 3 minutes per side, until deep golden brown, almost charred, using more oil as necessary. Transfer the wedges to one baking sheet, spaced slightly apart.

4. In a small bowl, whisk the lemon zest and juice, olive oil, garlic, salt, pepper, and pepper flakes. Baste each cabbage wedge generously, then pour the remaining mixture all over the cabbage. Roast the cabbage on the middle rack of the oven for 40 minutes, until softened at the core but crispy at the edges.

5. Meanwhile, transfer the tempeh from the marinade to the second baking sheet, evenly spacing the pieces; set the marinade aside.

6. After the cabbage has roasted for 15 minutes, place the tempeh on the bottom oven rack and roast for 10 minutes. Flip the pieces of tempeh and baste generously with the reserved marinade. Roast for another 8 to 10 minutes, until caramelized and crispy.

7. Plate the wedges of cabbage on a platter, crumble over the tempeh bacon, and sprinkle with the chives.

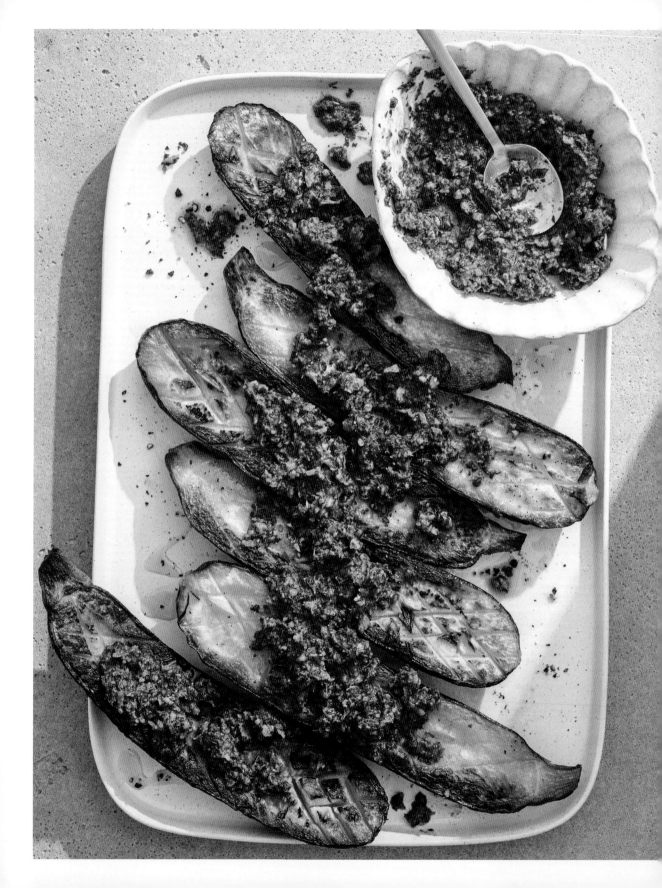

Pan-Roasted Zucchini with Lemony Herb Pesto

Serves: 4 to 6

Prep Time: 30 minutes, including salting the zucchini

Cook Time: 30 minutes

Zucchini

4 zucchini, halved lengthwise

½ teaspoon kosher salt

1 to 2 tablespoons avocado oil

Pesto

1 cup loosely packed fresh cilantro leaves and soft stems

1 cup loosely packed fresh flat-leaf parsley leaves and soft stems

1 green chile, seeded and roughly chopped

2 garlic cloves, peeled

⅓ cup raw almonds

1 tablespoon grated lemon zest

2 tablespoons lemon juice

2 tablespoons extra-virgin olive oil

2 teaspoons maple syrup (optional)

½ teaspoon kosher salt

¼ teaspoon ground black pepper

This is a great make-ahead side dish, as it can be served at room temperature. Roasting zucchini is a great way to bring out its flavors while still maintaining the integrity of its texture. I've topped it with a nutrient-rich pesto made from protein-packed almonds and fresh, bright herbs.

1. **For the zucchini:** Line a baking sheet with parchment paper. Arrange the zucchini halves cut side up, sprinkle with the salt, and let sit for 20 minutes. Pat dry with a paper towel.

2. Preheat the oven to 450°F.

3. Heat 1 tablespoon of the avocado oil in a large cast-iron pan or griddle over medium-high heat. Working in batches and adding more oil as necessary, add the zucchini, cut side down, and cook for 5 minutes, until golden; use a spatula to press the zucchini gently against the pan to ensure even cooking. Arrange the zucchini on the prepared baking sheet and roast for 20 to 25 minutes, until golden and softened.

4. **For the pesto:** Add the cilantro, parsley, chile, garlic, and almonds to a food processor and pulse until it resembles a crumb. Add the lemon zest and juice, 1 tablespoon of the olive oil, and the maple syrup, if using. Pulse a few more times, until the mixture comes together. Season with the salt and pepper. Transfer the pesto to a bowl and stir in the remaining 1 tablespoon olive oil.

5. Place the zucchini halves on a large platter, generously dollop nut pesto on top, and serve.

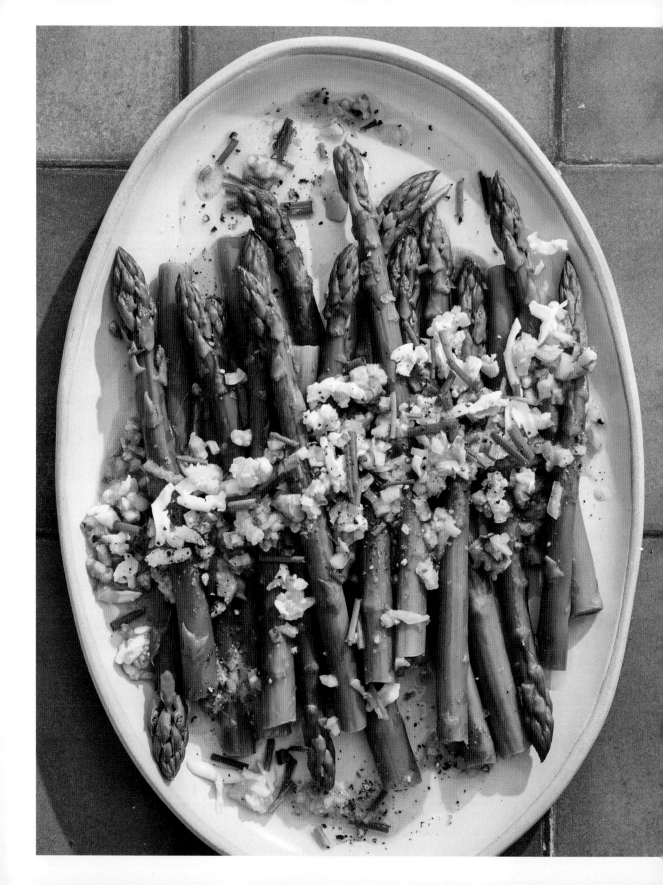

Asparagus Vinaigrette

Serves: 4 to 6

Prep Time: 15 minutes

Cook Time: 15 minutes

2 large pasture-raised organic eggs

1 pound asparagus, woody ends trimmed

1 large shallot, minced

1 tablespoon red wine vinegar

¼ cup extra-virgin olive oil

1 tablespoon water

1 garlic clove, grated

1 teaspoon Dijon mustard

1 teaspoon grainy Dijon mustard

1 teaspoon maple syrup

½ teaspoon kosher salt

Pinch of freshly ground black pepper, plus more for serving

2 tablespoons finely chopped toasted walnuts, for serving

1 tablespoon minced fresh chives, for serving

This take on a classic French dish uses beautiful bright green asparagus in place of the traditional leeks. Asparagus is packed with folate, an essential nutrient for healthy cell growth, as well as vitamin K, which is great for maintaining healthy bones. I've added some extra protein with omega-3-rich eggs, great for maintaining energy and brain health. Pair this side with grilled chicken or a firm white fish.

1. Bring a large pot of water to a boil over high heat. Add the eggs, reduce to a rolling boil, and cook for 9 minutes. Reserving the pot of boiling water, transfer the eggs to a large bowl of ice water and let cool for 5 minutes. Reserve the ice water, adding more ice if necessary.

2. Once the eggs are cool, peel, and use a box grater to grate them; set aside.

3. Add the asparagus to the boiling water and blanch over medium heat for 3 to 4 minutes, depending on the thickness of the stalks, until fork tender. Transfer with a slotted spoon to the bowl of ice water to stop the cooking. Once cool, transfer the asparagus to a paper towel–lined platter to dry.

4. In a small bowl, stir the shallot and vinegar together and let sit for 5 minutes. Add the olive oil, water, garlic, both mustards, maple syrup, salt, and pepper. Whisk until smooth.

5. Arrange the asparagus on a rimmed plate. Top with the dressing and sprinkle with the grated eggs. Add the toasted walnuts, chives, and a good crack of fresh black pepper.

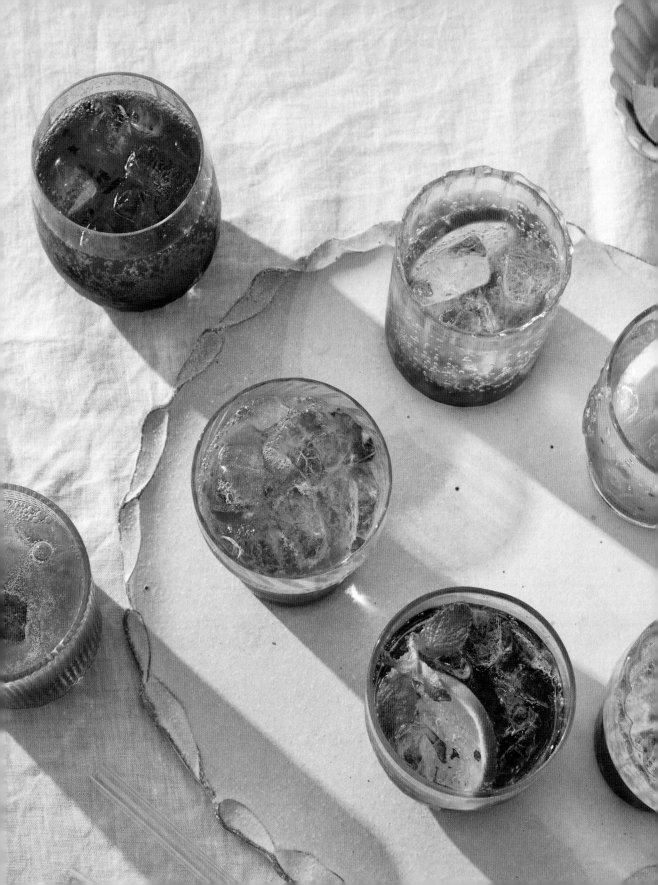

Drinks

There is something magical about creating your own health-promoting beverages at home. Drinks offer an opportunity to add color, flavor, and vibrancy to your day. Whether that means starting the day off with a glass of delicious homemade nut milk, pausing for a midday Matcha Vanilla Latte (page 170), or ending it with one of three Refresher mocktails (pages 171, 175, and 176), I believe drinks deserve a little more attention than they usually receive. Here, I show you how to make a variety of hot, cold, and much healthier beverages that are bound to become a new routine in your household.

Homemade Nut Milk

Makes: 4 cups

Prep Time: 30 minutes, plus at least 8 hours soaking

1 cup raw whole almonds

1 cup raw cashews

4 cups filtered water

½ cup unsweetened desiccated coconut (optional)

1 tablespoon maple syrup (optional)

Pinch of sea salt

Nuts often find their way into my cooking. Rich in healthy fats, vitamin E, omega-3s, and fiber, they are fundamental to our health. That's why I love to make my own nut milk that is pure, nutritious, creamy, and not filled with gums and oils like many store-bought milks. It takes a few steps to make, but once you try it in your coffee, smoothie, or any warm beverage, you'll be amazed at the intense flavor and texture.

It's important to first soak the nuts because it helps to germinate them, allowing the natural enzymes and nutrients to take hold. You'll need cheesecloth for straining the nut milk. Fresh nut milk will keep in a glass jar in the refrigerator for 4 days, or can be frozen in ice cube trays, then popped into your blender for smoothies or quickly defrosted for your morning latte.

1. Place the almonds and cashews in a large bowl and add enough water to cover. Soak in the refrigerator for at least 8 hours, or best overnight.

2. Drain and rinse the nuts. Working in batches, place half in a blender with 2 cups of the filtered water. Blend on high until smooth. Transfer to a large bowl. Repeat with the remaining nuts and 2 cups water, adding the coconut and maple syrup if using. Transfer the second batch to the bowl, mix to combine, and season with the salt.

3. Place cheesecloth over a large jug or bowl and carefully ladle or pour the milk over it. You will want to do this in batches, gathering the cheesecloth to squeeze out the milk as much as possible. (If you like, place the pulp left inside the cheesecloth in a bowl and set aside to freeze or make nut flour; see Tip.)

4. Pour the milk through a fine sieve into a glass mason jar. Cover with the lid and store in the refrigerator for 3 to 4 days.

Tip: *The wet nut pulp can be frozen and used for energy balls or in granola. Or make nut flour: Preheat the oven to 200°F. Line a baking sheet with parchment paper and spread the pulp evenly. Bake for 2 hours, stirring often, until it is as dry as possible. Place in a blender and blitz until a fine powder has formed. This can now be used like almond flour.*

Reishi Cacao Latte

Serves: 1

Prep Time: 5 minutes

1½ cups Homemade Nut Milk (page 166) or other nondairy milk

1 tablespoon raw unsweetened cacao powder

1 teaspoon reishi powder

½ teaspoon ground cinnamon

1 to 2 teaspoons maple syrup, to taste

This delicious latte is the healthier version of hot chocolate you didn't know you needed. Adaptogens are active ingredients found in mushrooms that provide many health benefits, like improved digestion, stress relief, improved immune function, and helping your body better respond to stress and anxiety. Reishi powder (made from reishi mushrooms) helps support the adrenal glands, which release cortisol, a hormone that helps your body respond to stress, as well as polysaccharides, which can help reduce inflammation.

Heat all the ingredients in a small saucepan over medium heat, whisking vigorously to dissolve the powders as the milk comes up to a simmer. Remove from the heat and serve.

Creamy Almond Masala Chai Latte

Serves: 2

Prep Time: 5 minutes

Chai Spice Mix

2 tablespoons ground cinnamon

1 tablespoon ground ginger

2 teaspoons ground cardamom

¼ teaspoon freshly ground black pepper

¼ teaspoon ground cloves

¼ teaspoon ground nutmeg

Chai Latte

1 tablespoon chai spice mix

2 cups macadamia nut milk

1 tablespoon smooth almond butter

1 tablespoon maple syrup

Masala chai is a fragrant spice blend known for its health benefits, such as improved digestion and heart health. With a mixture of warming spices—cinnamon, ginger, cardamom—it's delicious when blended with creamy macadamia milk and almond butter. I like to make the quick masala spice blend and keep it in a jar in my pantry, so I have it handy whenever I want to whip up this latte, add to a vanilla protein shake, or mix into the batter for my Trail-Mix Energy Cookies (page 183).

1. **For the chai spice mix:** Combine all the ingredients in an airtight container, mixing well.

2. **For the latte:** In a blender, combine 1 tablespoon of the chai spice mix and the remaining latte ingredients and blend until smooth. Pour over ice or gently heat on the stove until simmering.

3. Store the remaining chai spice mix in your pantry for up to 2 months for best flavor.

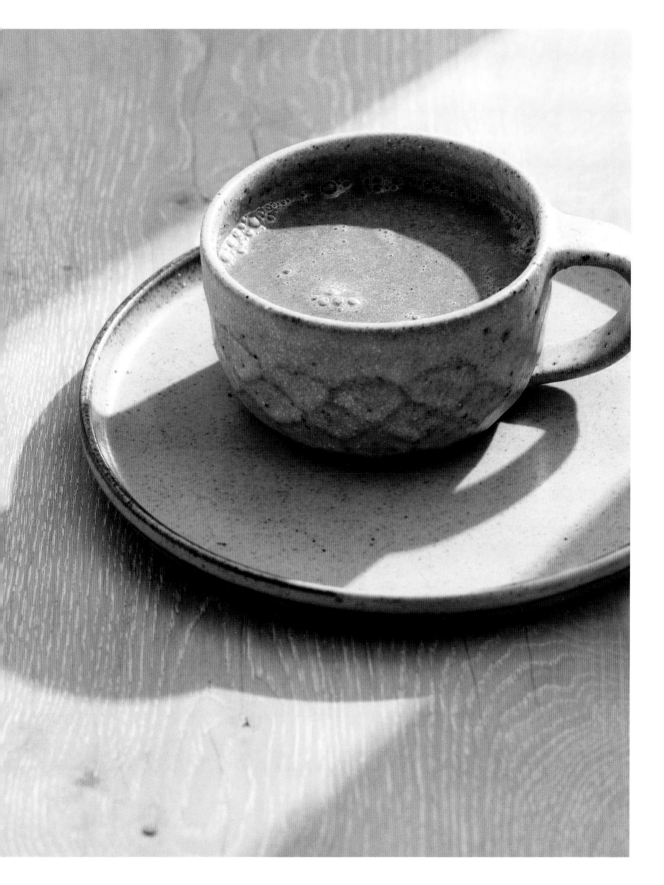

Matcha Vanilla Latte

Serves: 1

Prep Time: 5 minutes

1 cup Homemade Nut Milk
(page 166) or other nondairy milk

1 tablespoon collagen peptides
powder

1 teaspoon maple syrup

½ teaspoon matcha powder

½ teaspoon vanilla extract

Matcha is a great coffee alternative, and the perfect morning beverage. It's a potent green tea packed with nutrients and antioxidants as well as caffeine, for that morning boost. I've added powdered collagen not only for its creamy texture, but also for its powerful health benefits, like improved skin elasticity and joint-pain relief.

1. In a blender, combine all the ingredients. Blend until smooth and creamy.

2. Pour into a saucepan and bring to a simmer over medium heat. Remove and serve immediately.

Blackberry and Mint Refresher

Serves: 4

Prep Time: 15 minutes

1½ cups fresh blackberries, chopped

½ cup fresh lime juice

12 large fresh mint leaves

1 teaspoon monk fruit sweetener (optional)

Sparkling water, for serving

For this twist on the classic mojito, I've added fresh blackberries for sweetness and their vibrant hue. Blackberries are a superfood, filled with vitamins C and K and manganese, all of which help with bone health and building a strong immune system.

1. Divide the chopped berries among four glasses. Add 2 tablespoons lime juice to each glass along with two or three roughly torn mint leaves. Using a cocktail muddler, pound the berries and the mint until they release all their juices. Add sweetener if desired.

2. Fill each glass with ice and top with sparkling water. Garnish with extra mint, stir, and enjoy.

Iced Matcha Lemonade

Serves: 4

Prep Time: 40 minutes,
including chilling time

2 teaspoons matcha powder

2 cups boiling water

4 teaspoons maple syrup

½ cup lemon juice

Sparkling water (optional)

This is a refreshing caffeinated alternative to coffee in the summer months. The bitterness of antioxidant-rich green tea pairs well with the tangy, slightly sweetened lemonade. I like to top it off with sparkling water for an extra kick.

1. Place the matcha powder in a heatproof jug or bowl. While whisking, gradually pour in the just-boiled water and whisk until the matcha is fully dissolved. Refrigerate the matcha for at least 30 minutes, until chilled.

2. Divide the matcha among four glasses. Add 1 teaspoon maple syrup and 2 tablespoons lemon juice to each glass, stirring to combine. Fill each glass with ice and top with sparkling water, if desired.

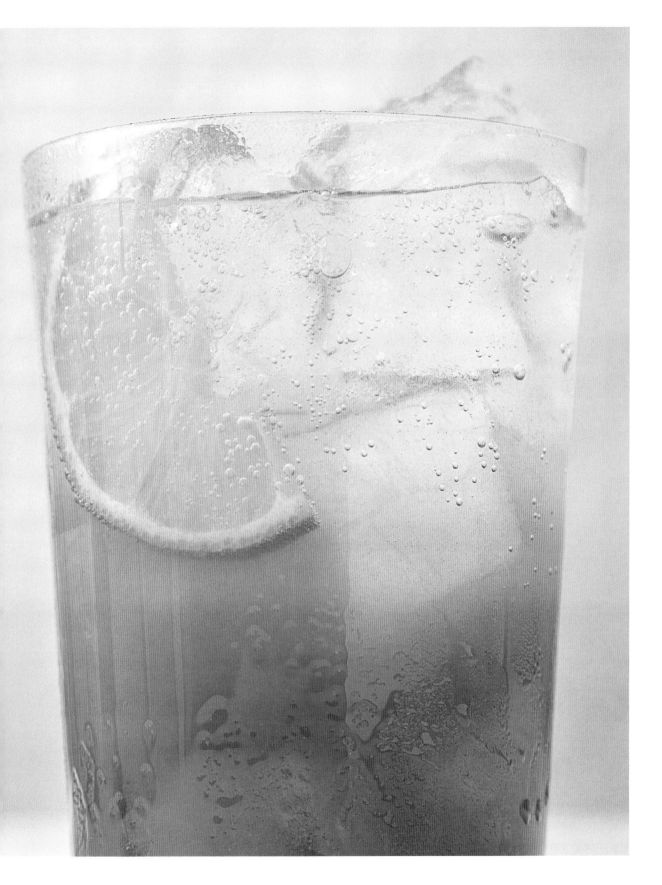

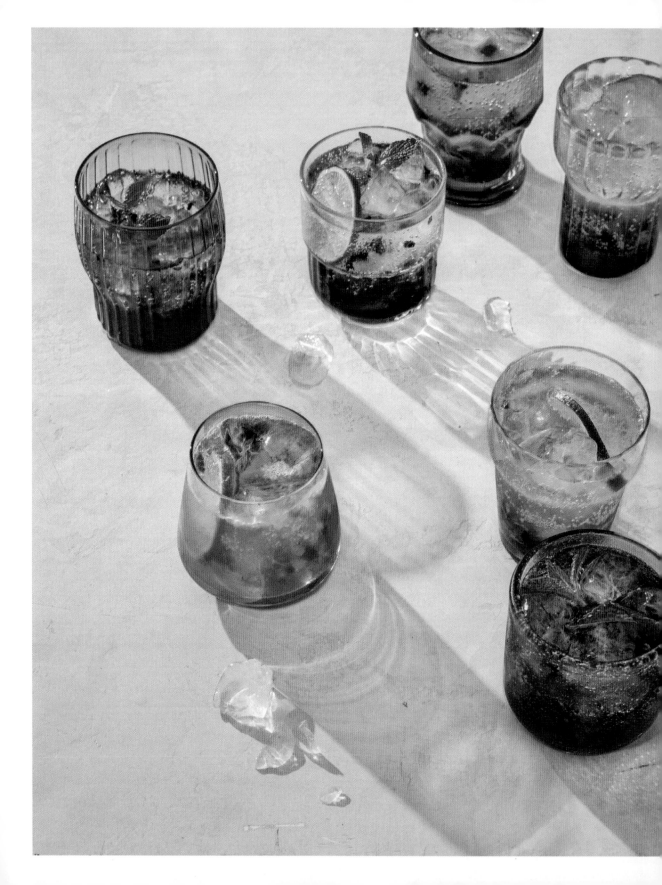

Strawberry and Basil Refresher

Serves: 4

Prep Time: 15 minutes

1 cup chopped strawberries

½ cup lime juice

12 large fresh basil leaves

1 teaspoon monk fruit sweetener (optional)

Sparkling water, for serving

This drink is best made with summer berries at peak ripeness that are oozing sweet juice. Strawberries are high in vitamin C and contain heart-healthy and cancer-fighting polyphenols. They also contain potassium, which can help maintain good blood pressure. Paired with herbaceous basil, this deliciously refreshing drink makes the perfect mocktail or after-noon spritz.

1. Divide the chopped berries among four glasses. Add 2 tablespoons lime juice to each glass along with two or three roughly torn basil leaves. Using a cocktail muddler, pound the berries and basil until they release all their juices. Add sweetener, if desired.

2. Fill each glass with ice and top with sparkling water. Garnish with extra basil, stir, and enjoy.

Hibiscus and Rose Refresher

Serves: 6 to 8

Prep Time: 1 hour, including chilling time

2 tablespoons hibiscus
tea leaves

4 cups boiling water

1 tablespoon maple syrup

¼ cup fresh lemon juice

2 teaspoons rosewater

Sparkling water, for serving

Hibiscus is a fruity, tangy flowering plant whose buds are perfect for tea. High in vitamin C and beta-carotene, antioxidant-rich hibiscus can provide a range of health benefits such as reducing inflammation and lowering blood pressure. Hibiscus tea is great chilled, and paired with floral notes from rosewater and bright lemon juice, it makes the perfect refreshing afternoon drink.

1. Place the hibiscus tea leaves in a heatproof jug, add the just-boiled water, and stir. Let steep for 5 minutes, then strain the tea into a pitcher. Add the maple syrup, stir, and chill in the refrigerator for at least 45 minutes. Add the lemon juice and rosewater.

2. Fill glasses about one-third full with the tea, then add ice. Top with sparkling water and serve.

Tulsi Tea Lemonade

Serves: 6

Prep Time: 1 hour, including chilling time

2 tablespoons tulsi tea leaves

4 cups boiling water

1 tablespoon maple syrup or honey

¼ cup lemon juice

Sparkling water, for serving

Tulsi, also known as holy basil, is a superfood rich in nutritional and therapeutic benefits. An ayurvedic adaptogen, tulsi tea contains ursolic acid, which promotes a sense of calm and can reduce stress and anxiety. This refreshing tea lemonade is perfect for an afternoon pick-me-up.

1. Place the tulsi tea leaves in a heatproof bowl, add the just-boiled water, and stir. Let steep for 5 minutes, then strain into a pitcher. Add the maple syrup or honey, stir, and chill in the refrigerator for at least 45 minutes, until chilled. Add the lemon juice.

2. Fill glasses with ice, then top off with the tea lemonade and a splash of sparkling water.

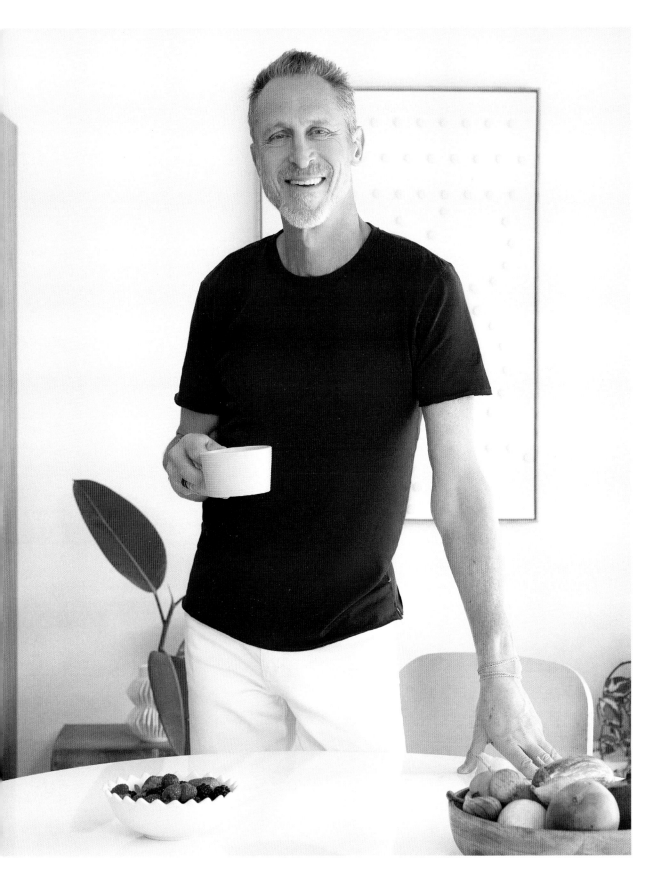

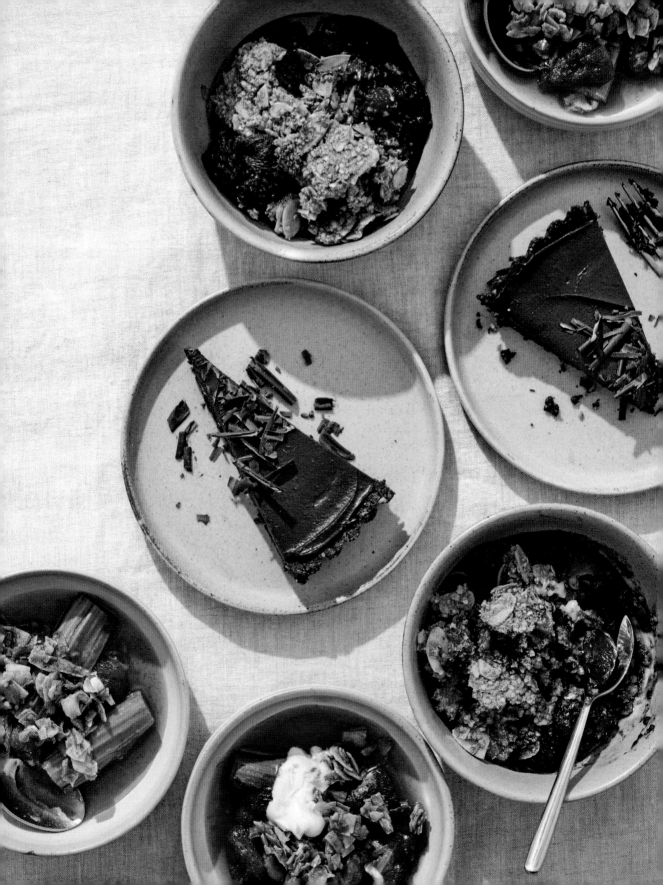

Desserts

I'll be the first to admit that I have a sweet tooth! And while moderation is key when it comes to desserts, there can be a way to indulge in decadent treats while still creating optimal health. Whether it's a slice of dairy-free cake or a bite of nori-flecked dark chocolate, there is something here for you. I especially love my gluten- and dairy-free

Chewy Chocolate Coconut Cookies (page 191) warm from the oven, or my puffed Quinoa, Cashew, and Dark Chocolate Squares (page 185) to help through the midafternoon slump. These thoughtfully created recipes are designed to add both nutrition and satisfaction, making them the perfect ending to any day.

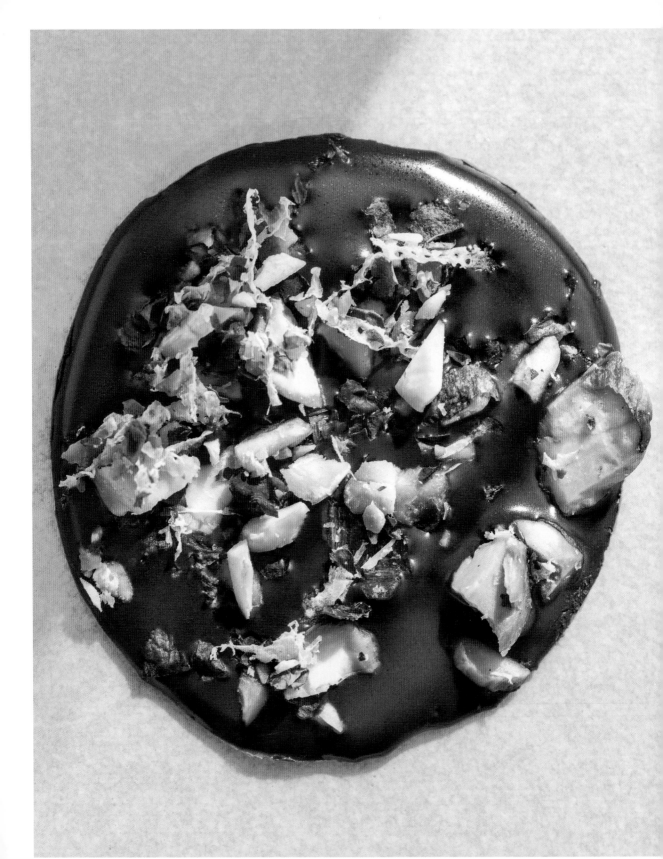

Dark Chocolate Seaweed Rounds

Makes: 20 rounds

Prep Time: 30 minutes,
including chilling time

Cook Time: 5 minutes

2 tablespoons finely chopped
raw pistachios

1 teaspoon green nori flakes

½ teaspoon finely grated
lemon zest

½ teaspoon flaky sea salt

6 ounces dark (70 percent cacao)
chocolate

1 teaspoon coconut oil

These umami dark chocolate rounds are a unique twist on an after-dinner treat. Both sweet and savory, the combination of delicate nori with bright lemon, pistachios, and salt makes these chocolate treats simply irresistible. Nori contains key nutrients like iodine, which helps regulate your thyroid, while dark chocolate contains flavonoids, which are helpful for the heart. The pistachios add a nutty flavor and a hit of plant-based protein, offering an added boost of nutrition.

1. Line a baking sheet with parchment paper and set aside.

2. In a bowl, combine the pistachios, nori flakes, lemon zest, and salt.

3. Place the chocolate and coconut oil in a heatproof bowl. Make a double boiler by filling a pot with 3 inches of water. Place over medium heat and bring to a simmer. Set the bowl of chocolate on top of the pot, but not touching the water, and gently melt the chocolate, stirring often. Once melted completely, carefully remove the bowl from the heat and allow it to cool slightly.

4. Using a spoon, drop about a quarter-sized amount of chocolate onto the baking sheet and sprinkle with some of the nori mixture. Repeat to make about 20 rounds. Chill the baking sheet in the fridge for at least 20 minutes. Store in an airtight container in the fridge for up to 2 weeks or in the freezer for up to 3 months.

Olive Oil and Almond Cake

Serves: 6 to 8

Prep Time: 20 minutes

Cook Time: 35 minutes

Almond Cake

2 cups fine-ground almond flour

1 teaspoon baking powder

¼ teaspoon kosher salt

3 large pasture-raised organic eggs, yolks and whites separated, at room temperature

¼ cup monk fruit sweetener

Grated zest of 1 orange

Grated zest of 1 lemon

⅓ cup extra-virgin olive oil, plus more for the pan

⅓ cup coconut yogurt

Orange Glaze

¼ cup monk fruit sweetener

2 to 3 tablespoons orange juice, strained

A simple cake that's not too sweet, loaded with goodness, and easy to make? I've got just the one for you. This olive oil–almond cake is gluten-free, dairy-free, and filled with flavor. Notes of bright citrus pair well with rich fruity extra-virgin olive oil and creamy almonds. Olive oil is extremely beneficial, providing ample healthy fats and antioxidants that help to combat oxidative stress, which over time can impair your brain health. I love to serve the cake with fresh fruit or, if I really want to indulge, a drizzle of melted dark chocolate.

1. Preheat the oven to 350°F. Lightly oil a 9x13-inch loaf pan and line with parchment paper.

2. For the cake: In a bowl, combine the almond flour, baking powder, and salt; set aside.

3. Using a stand mixer fitted with a whisk, or an electric hand mixer, whisk the egg yolks and sweetener together in a large bowl for 2 minutes, until slightly thickened. Add the orange zest, lemon zest, and olive oil and whisk until smooth. Fold in the almond flour mixture, alternating with the yogurt.

4. In a separate bowl, using a clean mixer, whisk the egg whites until they have thickened and doubled in volume, forming soft peaks.

5. Add one-third of the whites to the cake batter, stirring well until fully combined. Add the remaining whites very gently, folding them in.

6. Pour the batter into the prepared pan. Bake for 30 to 35 minutes, until golden and a cake tester comes out clean.

7. For the glaze: While the cake is baking, whisk the sweetener with the orange juice in a pan over medium heat for 3 to 5 minutes, until dissolved. Pour the glaze over the cake while it's warm, then allow the cake to cool completely before serving.

8. Store in a sealed container at room temperature for up to 3 days.

Trail-Mix Energy Cookies

Makes: 14 cookies

Prep Time: 30 minutes, including chilling time

Cook Time: 15 minutes

½ cup almond butter

¼ cup (½ stick) grass-fed unsalted butter, melted

¼ cup maple syrup

1 large pasture-raised organic egg, at room temperature

½ teaspoon ground cinnamon

¼ teaspoon kosher salt

1 cup almond flour

½ teaspoon baking powder

½ teaspoon baking soda

½ cup roughly chopped walnuts

⅓ cup pumpkin seeds

⅓ cup roughly chopped whole almonds

⅓ cup dried cherries or cranberries

These energizing cookies are crammed with wholesome trail-mix favorites—nuts, seeds, dried fruit—and perfect for when you're on the go. A great source of protein, fiber, and healthy fats, they use almond flour, a gluten-free, nutrient-dense flour alternative. I love to make a double batch and freeze half, so I always have some ready to take with me when I'm hiking or out for the day.

1. Preheat the oven to 350°F. Line a baking sheet with parchment paper.

2. In a large bowl, whisk the almond butter, butter, maple syrup, and egg together until smooth. Whisk in the cinnamon and salt.

3. Add the almond flour, baking powder, and baking soda and stir until fully combined. Stir in the walnuts, pumpkin seeds, almonds, and dried fruit. Chill the batter for at least 15 minutes.

4. Scoop up heaping tablespoons of dough and roll into balls. Flatten the balls on the baking sheet. Bake for 13 to 15 minutes, until the cookies are puffed and golden. Allow to cool slightly before serving.

5. Store in an airtight container up to 1 week.

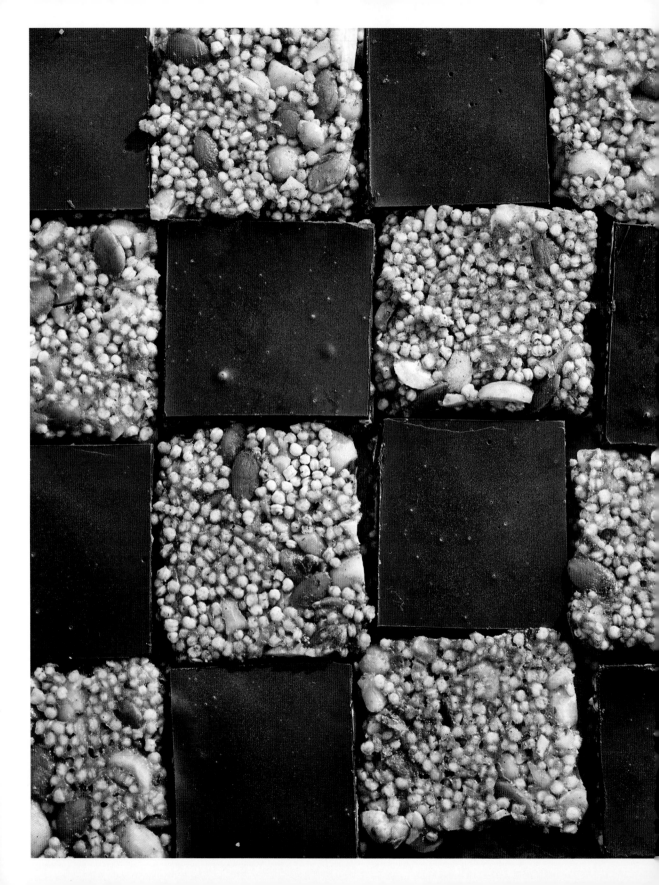

Quinoa, Cashew, and Dark Chocolate Squares

Makes: 16 squares

Prep Time: 45 minutes, including chilling time

Cook Time: 5 minutes

Quinoa and Cashew Squares

½ cup pitted Medjool dates

½ cup cashew butter

½ cup water

1 tablespoon coconut oil

½ teaspoon vanilla extract

½ teaspoon ground cinnamon

2½ cups puffed quinoa

1 cup roughly chopped cashews

¼ cup pumpkin seeds

Chocolate Glaze

5 ounces dark (70 percent cacao) chocolate

1 tablespoon coconut oil

These cashew butter bites are a great, energizing treat to stash in the fridge for when you need a hit of something sweet. A base of puffed quinoa, loaded with nuts and seeds and topped with a layer of dark chocolate, is the perfect combination of texture and flavor that won't make your blood sugar spike. Cashews are rich in fiber, protein, and heart-healthy monounsaturated fats like oleic and palmitoleic acids. They are super creamy, and, when paired with dates, they almost taste like caramel!

1. Line an 8x8-inch square pan with plastic wrap.

2. **For the squares:** In a pot over medium heat, combine the dates, cashew butter, water, coconut oil, vanilla, and cinnamon. Cover and cook for 1 minute. Transfer the mixture to a food processor and blend until smooth.

3. Using a spatula, scrape the date mixture into a large bowl and fold in the puffed quinoa, cashews, and pumpkin seeds until well combined. Transfer to the prepared pan and flatten until smooth, pressing down firmly. Freeze for 20 minutes, until firm.

4. **For the glaze:** Combine the chocolate and coconut oil in a heatproof bowl. Make a double boiler by filling a pot with 3 inches of water. Place over medium heat and bring to a simmer. Set the bowl of chocolate on top of the pot, but not touching the water, and gently melt the chocolate, stirring often. Once melted completely, carefully remove the bowl from the heat and allow it to cool slightly.

5. Pour the chocolate over the cashew mixture, tilting the pan until it is an even layer. Refrigerate for another 20 minutes, until firm.

6. Remove from the tin and discard the plastic wrap. Cut into 16 squares. Store in an airtight container in the refrigerator for up to 2 weeks.

Coconut and Chocolate Blueberry Clusters

Makes: 20

Prep Time: 30 minutes, including chilling time

Cook Time: 5 minutes

6 ounces dark (70 percent cacao) chocolate

1 tablespoon coconut oil

1 cup fresh blueberries

½ cup toasted coconut chips

I keep these in my fridge or freezer for when I'm craving something fruity but with a bit more substance. You can easily make them with any berry and/or swap out the coconut for nuts or seeds. I like to use blueberries because not only do they pair perfectly with chocolate, they are high in phytochemicals that promote good gut health and reduce inflammation.

1. Place the chocolate and coconut oil in a heatproof bowl. Make a double boiler by filling a pot with 3 inches of water. Place over medium heat and bring to a simmer. Set the bowl of chocolate on top of the pot, but not touching the water, and gently melt the chocolate, stirring often. Once melted completely, carefully remove the bowl from the heat and allow it to cool slightly.

2. Using a spoon, drop quarter-sized portions of chocolate onto the baking sheet. Top each with three blueberries and some coconut chips. Drizzle a bit of chocolate over the blueberries. Chill the baking sheet in the fridge for at least 20 minutes.

3. Store in an airtight container in the fridge for up to 2 weeks or in the freezer for up to 3 months.

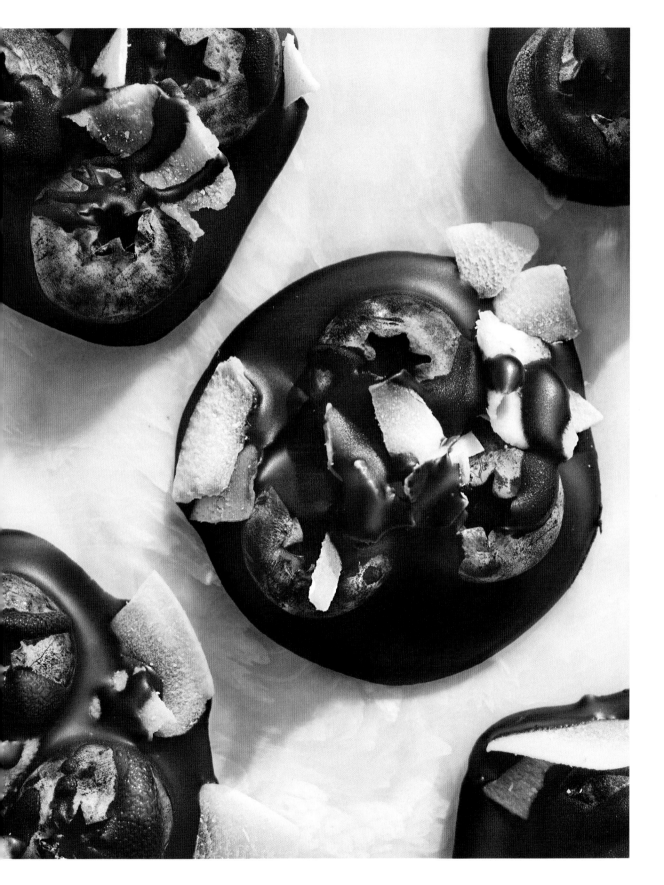

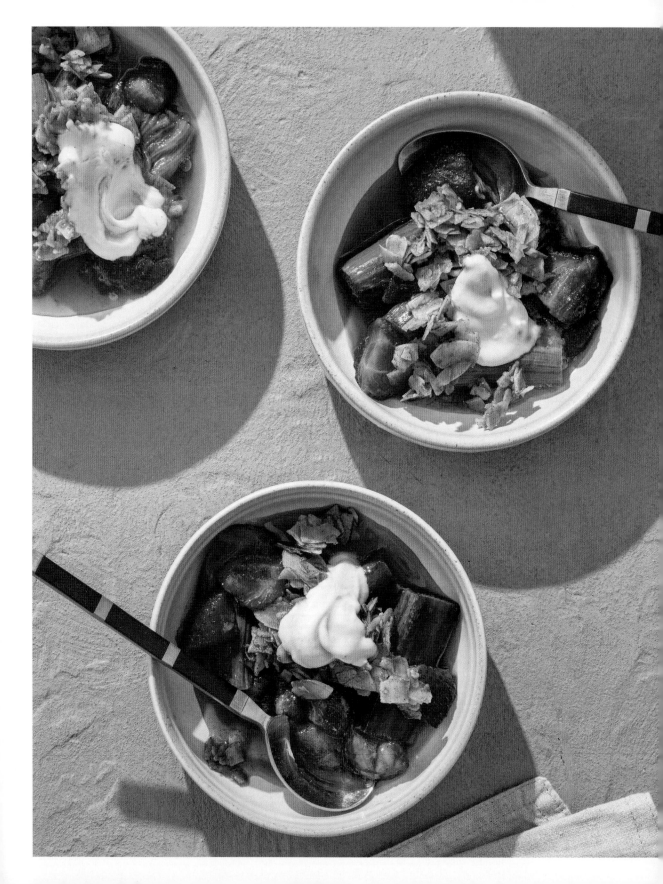

Roasted Rhubarb-Strawberry Coconut Crumble

Serves: 4 to 6

Prep Time: 20 minutes

Cook Time: 25 minutes

Rhubarb and Strawberries

2 pounds rhubarb, cut into 2½-inch pieces

2 cups strawberries, halved

¾ cup monk fruit sweetener

1 teaspoon grated lemon zest

2 teaspoons lemon juice

1 teaspoon vanilla extract

Coconut Crumble

1 cup unsweetened coconut flakes

½ teaspoon ground cinnamon

2 tablespoons honey or maple syrup, warmed

Coconut Cream

1 (13.5-ounce) can full-fat unsweetened coconut milk, chilled for at least 3 hours

½ teaspoon vanilla extract

1 tablespoon monk fruit sweetener

Rhubarb is a unique springtime vegetable, with the most beautiful vibrant pink stems, that lends itself well to both sweet and savory pairings. Naturally sour, you need to add a sweetener to make rhubarb pleasant to eat, but once it's roasted in the oven alongside sweet strawberries, you'll realize the true potential of this delicious veggie. Served with whipped coconut cream and a crunchy coconut crumble topping, this dessert is an elevated pairing, perfect for entertaining.

1. Preheat the oven to 400°F.

2. **For the rhubarb and strawberries:** Combine the rhubarb and strawberries in a roasting pan with the sweetener, lemon zest, lemon juice, and vanilla. Mix well and cover the pan with foil. Bake for 15 to 20 minutes, until softened. Remove the foil and continue baking for 5 minutes, until the liquid thickens and becomes syrupy.

3. **For the coconut crumble:** Place the coconut flakes in a large nonstick pan and toast over medium heat for about 5 minutes, stirring frequently. Add the cinnamon, then the honey or maple syrup and stir to mix well. Remove from the heat and let cool completely.

4. **For the coconut cream:** Scoop the thick coconut cream from the top of the can and place in a large bowl. (The remaining coconut milk can be refrigerated and used for smoothies or cooking.) Add the vanilla and sweetener to the coconut cream and beat with an electric mixer until thickened and smooth with the texture of whipped cream.

5. Scoop the rhubarb and strawberries into bowls, top with coconut cream and some crunchy coconut crumble, and serve.

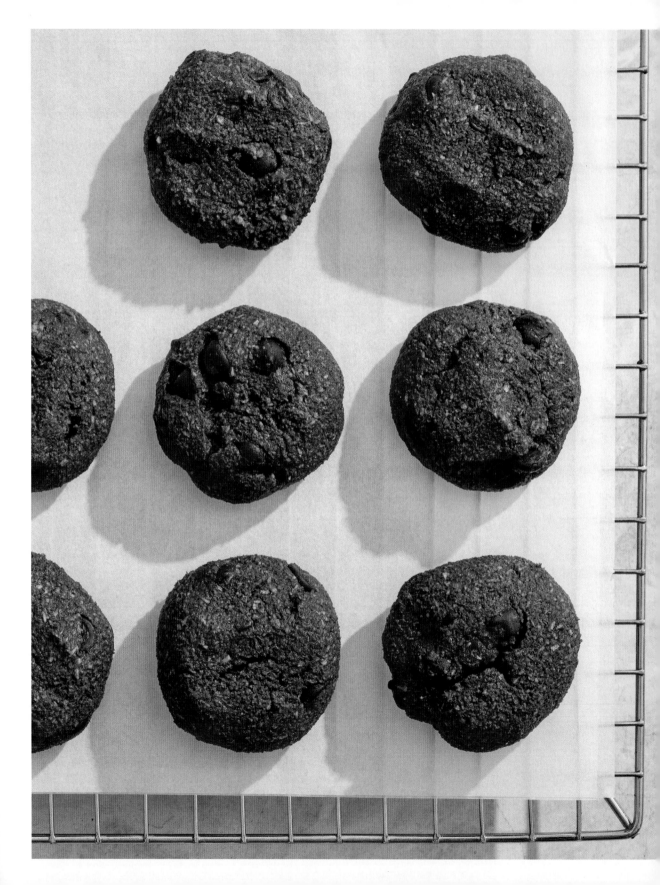

Chewy Chocolate Coconut Cookies

Makes: 14
Prep Time: 35 minutes,
including chilling time
Cook Time: 15 minutes

1 cup almond flour

½ cup unsweetened
shredded coconut

¼ cup unsweetened raw
cacao powder

2 tablespoons arrowroot powder

¼ teaspoon kosher salt

2 large pasture-raised
organic eggs

⅓ cup maple syrup

2 tablespoons coconut oil, melted

½ cup dark (70 percent cacao)
chocolate chips

You would never guess these cookies are gluten-free—they are that good! Crispy on the outside, chewy in the center, chocolate coconut cookies will satisfy any craving.

1. Preheat the oven to 350°F. Line a baking sheet with parchment paper.

2. In a large bowl, combine the almond flour, coconut, cacao powder, arrowroot powder, and salt. In a small bowl, whisk the eggs, maple syrup, and coconut oil.

3. Pour the egg mixture into the flour mixture and stir until well combined. Add the chocolate chips and stir. Refrigerate for at least 20 minutes, until slightly firm.

4. Scoop up heaping tablespoons of dough and roll into balls. Flatten the balls slightly onto the baking sheet. Bake for 15 minutes, until puffed and crispy. Allow to cool completely.

5. Store in an airtight container in the fridge for up to 2 weeks.

Tip: *The dough balls can easily be made ahead and frozen in an airtight container. Adjust the baking time slightly if baking from frozen (or allow them to thaw slightly before baking).*

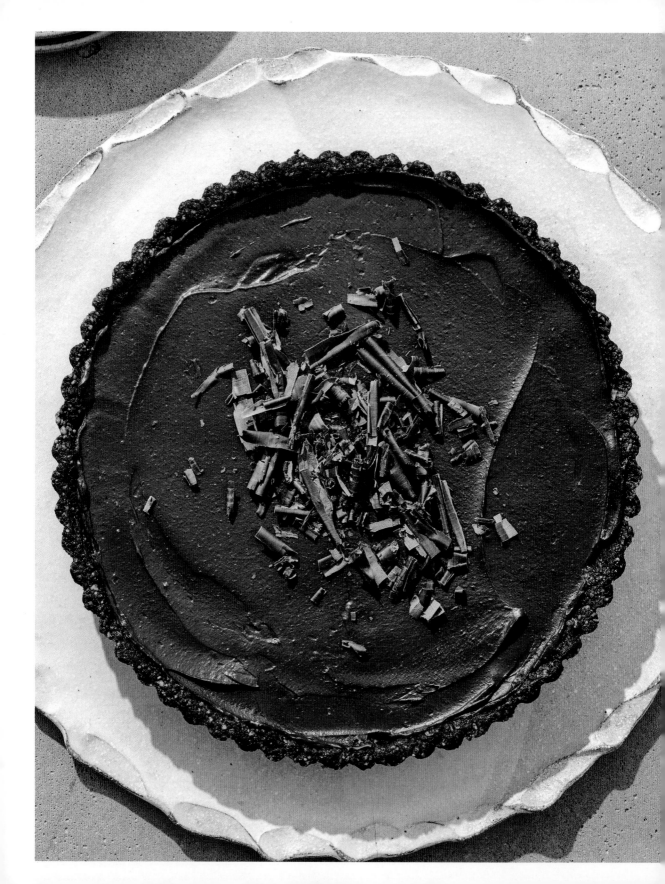

Raw Chocolate Tart

Serves: 8 to 10

Prep Time: 20 minutes,
plus 2½ hours chilling

Nut Base

1 cup raw Brazil nuts

1 cup raw walnuts

4 ounces pitted Medjool dates

4 ounces dried figs

¼ cup unsweetened raw
cacao powder

2 tablespoons coconut oil,
melted

Filling

2 medium ripe avocados,
pitted and peeled

½ cup maple syrup

¼ cup coconut oil, melted

1 tablespoon smooth almond
butter

½ teaspoon vanilla extract

⅓ cup unsweetened raw
cacao powder

½ teaspoon ground cinnamon

Chocolate shavings, for garnish

This show-stopping chocolate tart may look fancy, but it's easy enough for any beginner to make. It's a no-bake treat with both elements made in a food processor. The base is packed with nutrition and flavor from Brazil nuts, walnuts, dates, and dried figs. Brazil nuts are nutritional powerhouses, loaded with polyphenols and minerals like selenium, which helps with thyroid function and brain health. The rich chocolate filling is made with avocados, which contain heart-healthy omega-3 fats, and almond butter, providing a good dose of protein and fiber. The tart can be made in advance and refrigerated for up to 3 days.

1. Prepare a 9-inch round tart tin with a removable base by lining with a piece of plastic wrap so it hangs over all sides by at least 1 inch.

2. **For the nut base:** In a food processor, combine the Brazil nuts and walnuts and pulse a few times. Add the dates and figs and pulse again, until the mixture begins to come together. Add the cacao powder and coconut oil and pulse until well combined and the mixture sticks together when pressed between your fingers. Transfer the mixture to the prepared tart tin and press it onto the bottom and up the sides. Refrigerate for at least 30 minutes, until firm.

3. **For the filling:** Wipe the food processor clean. Add the avocados, maple syrup, coconut oil, almond butter, vanilla, cacao powder, and cinnamon. Blitz until smooth and fluffy. Transfer the mixture to the prepared tart base and smooth it out with the back of a spoon. Chill until firm, about 2 hours.

4. Remove the tart from the fridge 30 minutes prior to serving. Remove from the tin and garnish with chocolate shavings.

Coconut Matcha Popsicles

Makes: 6 to 8

Prep Time: 5 minutes,
plus freezing

1 (13.5-ounce) can full-fat
unsweetened coconut milk

½ cup nondairy milk

1 tablespoon matcha powder

2 to 3 tablespoons maple
syrup, to taste

These quick popsicles taste like a delicious matcha latte! Coconut and matcha are a delicious, refreshing combination because the creamy coconut offsets the slight bitterness of the green tea. A potent form of green tea, matcha is known for its high antioxidant properties, which can reduce inflammation and improve immune function. The superfood also contains caffeine and the amino acid L-theanine, which is known to reduce stress and anxiety. Make these to keep cool when the summer temperatures rise.

1. In a blender, combine all the ingredients and blend until smooth. Pour into popsicle molds and freeze overnight. Popsicles will keep frozen for up to 1 month.

2. Run the molds under hot water for 1 to 2 minutes to release the popsicles.

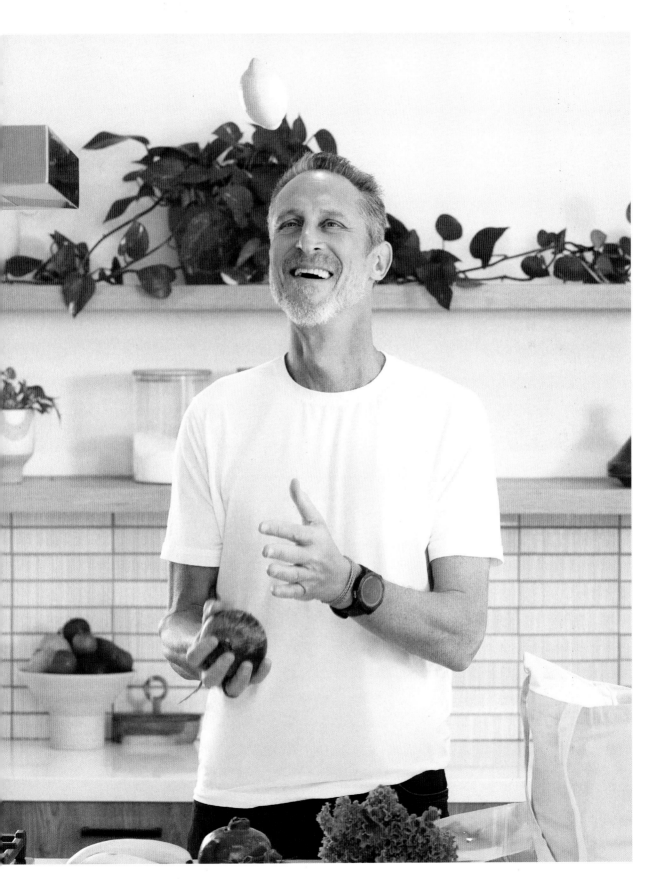

Mixed Berry and Almond Crisp

Serves: 6 to 8

Prep Time: 15 minutes

Cook Time: 25 minutes

Berry Filling

3 pounds mixed berries, such as blueberries, blackberries, raspberries, or strawberries (quartered if large)

2 tablespoons arrowroot powder

1 tablespoon lemon juice

1 teaspoon vanilla extract

1 to 2 tablespoons maple syrup, to taste

Crisp Topping

1¾ cups quinoa flakes

½ cup almond flour

1 cup sliced almonds, roughly chopped

1 teaspoon ground cinnamon

¼ cup maple syrup

¾ cup (1½ sticks) grass-fed unsalted butter or coconut oil, melted

½ cup unsweetened coconut yogurt, for serving (optional)

There is nothing like the sweet smell of a warm fruit crisp baking in the oven. Rich with summer berries and a crunchy crumble topping piled over the mound of bubbling fruit, this crisp is a delicious one-pan bake. Rich in the phytonutrient resveratrol, the antioxidant-filled berries help protect your body from AGEs (advanced glycation end products), a biomarker implicated in aging and degenerative disease. You can easily substitute other seasonal fruit.

1. Preheat the oven to 375°F.

2. **For the berry filling:** In a large bowl, combine all the ingredients. Transfer the mixture to a 12-inch ovenproof skillet.

3. **For the crisp topping:** In a large bowl, combine the quinoa flakes, almond flour, almonds, and cinnamon. Add the maple syrup and melted butter or coconut oil and stir until the mixture is no longer dry.

4. Crumble the topping all over the fruit. Bake for 25 minutes, until the berries are soft and bubbling and the topping is golden brown.

5. Scoop the berry crisp into bowls and top with dollops of yogurt if desired.

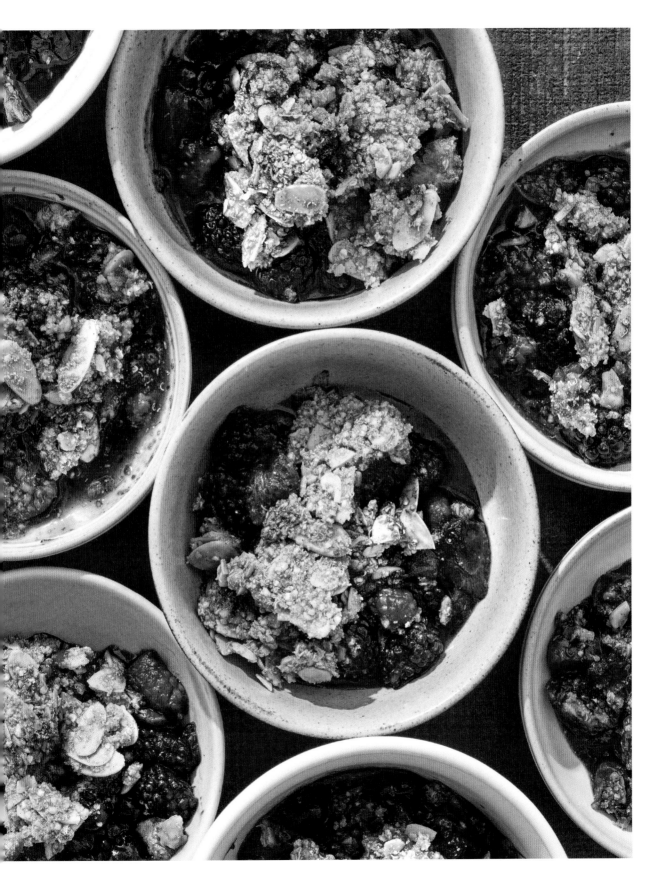

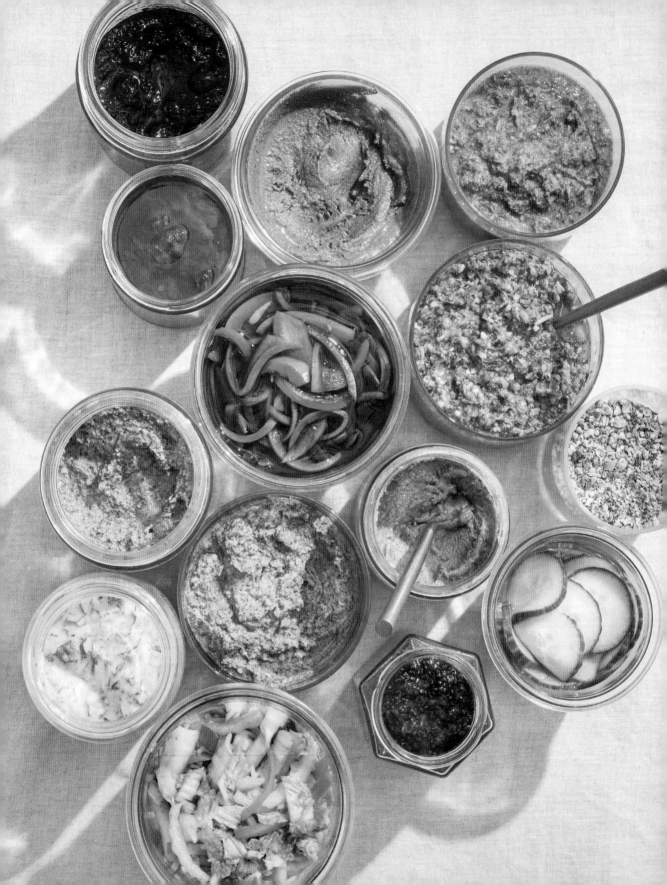

Condiments and Staples

This chapter is arguably one of the most important in the book. It provides quick ways to enhance your cooking: flavorful concoctions that can be whipped up in no time to add an explosion of textures, colors, and flavors to any meal. Pickled Red Onions (page 210) provide a bright tangy and sweet flavor that easily jazzes up eggs, salads, or roast chicken. If you're looking to be adventurous, try my variations on homemade pesto: Swap out the traditional pine nuts for omega-3-rich walnuts in my Basil Walnut Pesto (page 203); pair my Pistachio Mint Pesto (page 201) with your favorite grilled meats or veggies; or whip up my zesty Arugula and Pumpkin Seed Pesto (page 202), which is packed with antioxidants. You might also want to try out one of my easy chia jams (pages 217 and 219) for a low-sugar, protein-rich addition to your breakfast. There are a multitude of ways to tap into more flavorful cooking at home, and these recipes are a surefire way to do so.

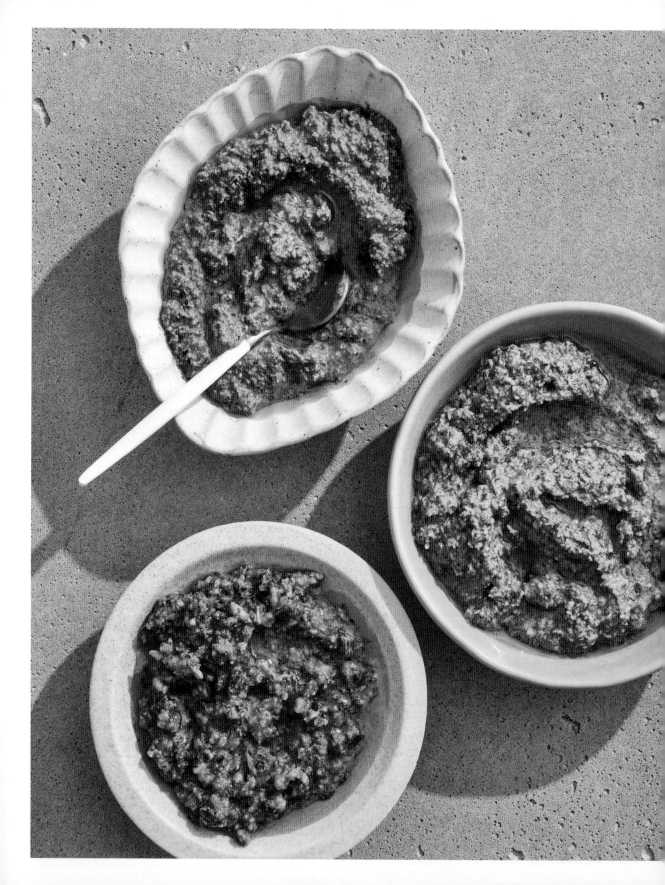

Pistachio Mint Pesto

Makes: 1½ cups

Prep Time: 10 minutes

1 cup toasted pistachios

2 garlic cloves, peeled

2 cups packed fresh mint leaves

½ cup fresh basil leaves

¼ cup lemon juice

⅔ cup extra-virgin olive oil

1 teaspoon kosher salt

Rich in flavor and nutrition, this pesto is simple and tasty. Pistachios are rich in vitamin B_6 and potassium, supporting blood sugar regulation and red blood cell formation. They also contain high levels of lutein, important for eye health. Serve the flavorful pesto alongside grilled meat or my Spice-Roasted Leg of Lamb (page 106).

1. In a food processor, pulse the pistachios and garlic until the nuts are a coarse texture. Add the mint and basil and continue pulsing until the mixture is roughly chopped. Add the lemon juice, half the olive oil, and salt. Pulse a few more times until the mixture comes together. Be careful not to overmix.

2. Transfer the pesto to a small bowl and stir in the remaining olive oil. Adjust the seasoning, if necessary.

3. Store in an airtight container in the refrigerator for up to 1 week or freeze for up to 2 months.

Arugula and Pumpkin Seed Pesto

Makes: 1 cup

Prep Time: 10 minutes

3 cups packed baby arugula

½ cup toasted pumpkin seeds

1 garlic clove, peeled

⅓ cup extra-virgin olive oil

2 tablespoons lemon juice

½ teaspoon kosher salt

¼ teaspoon freshly ground black pepper

Arugula packs a bright, peppery punch in this delicious pumpkin seed pesto. If you use regular arugula, you may need to adjust the amount of lemon juice to cut through the peppery flavor, but baby arugula works just fine! This antioxidant-rich pesto is the perfect spread or addition to any marinade.

1. In a food processor, combine the arugula, pumpkin seeds, and garlic. Pulse a few times, then add the olive oil, lemon juice, salt, and pepper. Blend until almost smooth.

2. Store in an airtight container in the refrigerator for up to 1 week or freeze for up to 2 months.

Basil Walnut Pesto

Makes: 1½ cups

Prep Time: 10 minutes

4 cups packed fresh basil leaves

1 cup toasted walnuts

1 garlic clove, peeled

½ cup extra-virgin olive oil

¼ cup lemon juice

⅓ cup grated pecorino cheese

½ teaspoon kosher salt

¼ teaspoon freshly ground black pepper

I love walnuts as they're rich in antioxidants as well as omega-3 fats, which can lower your risk of heart disease. They are also delicious when roasted and pair well with fresh basil for a twist on classic pesto. Use this pesto as a marinade for grilled chicken, a spread on a sandwich, or a sauce for roasted vegetables.

1. In a food processor, combine the basil, walnuts, and garlic. Pulse a few times before adding the olive oil, lemon juice, pecorino cheese, salt, and pepper. Blend until almost smooth.

2. Store in an airtight container in the refrigerator for up to 1 week or freeze for up to 2 months.

Cashew Hollandaise

Makes: 2 cups

Prep Time: 15 minutes

1 cup raw cashews

Boiling water

1 cup water

¼ cup lemon juice

2 tablespoons nutritional yeast

1 teaspoon Dijon mustard

1 teaspoon turmeric powder

½ teaspoon garlic powder

½ teaspoon kosher salt

This creamy and decadent nut-based hollandaise is a much healthier version of the traditional sauce. Made from cashew nuts and nutritional yeast, it's naturally gluten- and dairy-free. Cashews are packed with healthy fats and fiber, and they keep you feeling fuller, longer. They are also associated with a lower risk for age-related chronic disease and can improve your life span if consumed daily.

1. Place the cashews in a heatproof bowl and cover with just boiled water. Allow to soften for 10 minutes, then drain.

2. Transfer to a high-speed blender, add the 1 cup water and the remaining ingredients, and blend until smooth.

3. Store in an airtight container in the fridge for up to 4 days.

Salsa Verde

Makes: 1½ cups

Prep Time: 10 minutes

1 tablespoon Dijon mustard

4 anchovy fillets

1 garlic clove, peeled

2 cups fresh flat-leaf
parsley leaves

1 cup fresh basil leaves

1 cup fresh mint leaves

¼ cup fresh oregano leaves

2 tablespoons capers

1 teaspoon grated lemon zest

¼ cup lemon juice

1 tablespoon sherry or
red wine vinegar

½ cup extra-virgin olive oil

½ teaspoon kosher salt

½ teaspoon freshly ground
black pepper

Pinch of red pepper flakes

My version of salsa verde is a mash-up between chimichurri and traditional salsa verde. A mixture of fresh herbs, briny capers, sharp acid, and anchovy, it's the perfect condiment to jazz up any meal. Serve the bright sauce alongside your favorite grilled fish, meat, or vegetable.

1. In a food processor, combine the mustard, anchovies, and garlic and pulse a few times. Add the parsley, basil, mint, oregano, capers, lemon zest and juice, and vinegar and pulse until the mixture is finely chopped.

2. Add ¼ cup of the olive oil, the salt, pepper, and pepper flakes. Pulse until the mixture comes together. Transfer to a bowl and stir in the remaining ¼ cup olive oil.

3. Store in an airtight container in the refrigerator for up to 1 week or freeze for up to 2 months.

Chermoula

Makes: 1½ cups

Prep Time: 10 minutes

1 cup sheep's milk yogurt

3 tablespoons extra-virgin olive oil

1 cup loosely packed fresh cilantro leaves and soft stems, finely chopped

1 cup loosely packed fresh flat-leaf parsley leaves and soft stems, finely chopped

1 teaspoon grated lemon zest

2 tablespoons lemon juice

1 garlic clove, grated

2 teaspoons toasted cumin seeds

½ teaspoon red pepper flakes

½ teaspoon kosher salt

Pinch of freshly ground black pepper, to taste

This condiment has its origins in North African cuisine and is traditionally paired with seafood and meat. I've added creamy sheep's milk yogurt to cut the heat from the chili flakes and add additional texture to this delicious sauce.

1. In a bowl, whisk the yogurt, olive oil, cilantro, parsley, lemon zest and juice, garlic, cumin seeds, and red pepper flakes. Season with salt and pepper to taste.

2. Store in an airtight container in the fridge for up to 5 days.

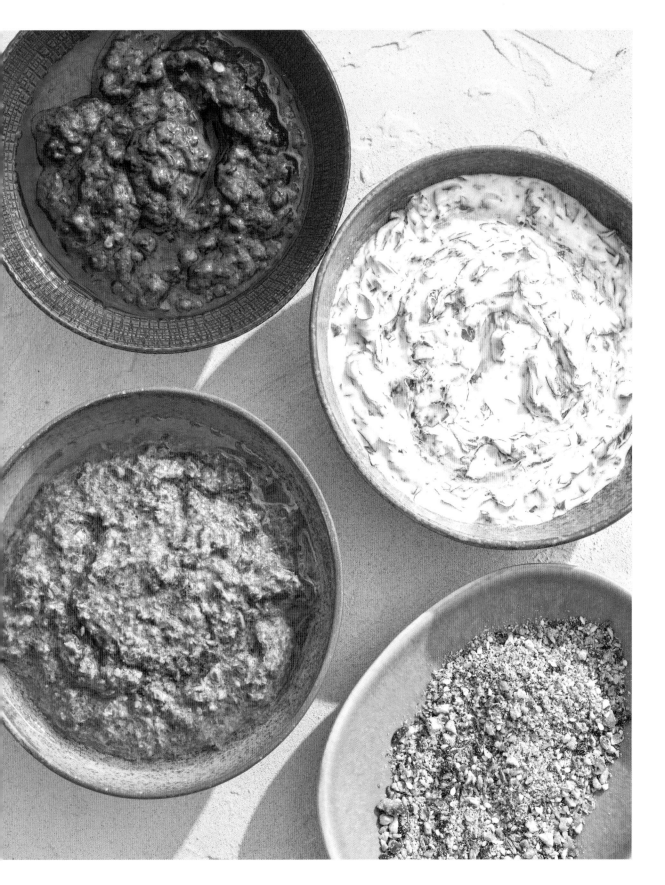

Harissa

Makes: ¾ cup

Prep Time: 35 minutes

Cook Time: 5 minutes

1 red bell pepper

1 teaspoon avocado oil

2 teaspoons coriander seeds

1 teaspoon cumin seeds

1 teaspoon caraway seeds

2 tablespoons paprika

1 teaspoon red pepper flakes

3 garlic cloves, peeled

1 teaspoon kosher salt

2 tablespoons extra-virgin olive oil, plus more for storing

Harissa is an easy-to-make paste that can be used to brighten sauces and marinades, stirred into yogurt, or simply served as a dip. Packed with delicious and nutritious spices like caraway and cumin, which promote good digestion, the pepper-chile paste is a great addition to your pantry. Instead of grilling a red pepper, you can use 1 roasted red pepper from a jar, drained.

1. Preheat the grill to 450°F. Lightly coat the red pepper with the avocado oil and roast on the grill, rotating until the skin is blackened all over, about 25 minutes. Place in a bowl and cover tightly with plastic wrap so the pepper can steam. Once cool enough to handle, peel the skin, open the pepper, and remove and discard the seeds.

2. In a small bowl, combine the coriander seeds, cumin seeds, and caraway seeds. Spread the spices out in a dry pan and toast on the stovetop over medium heat for 1 to 2 minutes, until fragrant; set aside to cool. Stir in the paprika and red pepper flakes.

3. Using a food processor, process the garlic cloves until they become a paste, then add the red pepper. Season with salt, add the spice mix and the olive oil, and blend well. Transfer the harissa to a lidded jar and cover with more olive oil to store.

4. Harissa will keep well in an airtight container in the fridge for 1 to 2 weeks or frozen up to 2 months.

Almond Dukkah

Makes: 1 cup

Prep Time: 15 minutes

Cook Time: 5 minutes

½ cup whole raw almonds

2 tablespoons sesame seeds

1 tablespoon coriander seeds

1 tablespoon cumin seeds

1 tablespoon fennel seeds

1 teaspoon black peppercorns

½ teaspoon flaky salt

Dukkah is an Egyptian nut and spice blend that adds bright flavor and texture to dishes. Crunchy, aromatic, and versatile, this condiment is a great topper to vegetables, dips, salads, and more.

1. Preheat the oven to 350°F. Place the almonds on a baking sheet and roast for 8 to 10 minutes, until toasted and golden. Allow to cool slightly.

2. Meanwhile, in a dry pan over medium heat, toast the sesame seeds, coriander seeds, cumin seeds, fennel seeds, and peppercorns, stirring often, until fragrant and golden, 1 to 2 minutes. Allow to cool slightly.

3. Place the roasted almonds and toasted spices in a food processor and add the salt. Pulse until the mixture resembles a fine crumb.

4. Allow the mixture to cool completely before storing in an airtight container in your pantry for up to 1 month.

Pickled Red Onions

**Makes: 4 cups,
including pickling juice**
Prep Time: 1 hour,
including cooling time
Cook Time: 5 minutes

1 cup red wine or apple cider
vinegar

¼ cup water

1 tablespoon kosher salt

2 cups thinly sliced red onions

One of my favorite condiments to keep stashed in the fridge, pickled onions go great with just about anything. Eggs, fish, chicken, salad—you name it. Quick and simple to make, they add the most wonderful bright, acidic note to any meal.

1. Combine the vinegar, water, and salt in a small saucepan and bring to a boil over medium heat.

2. Place the onions in a heatproof bowl and add the vinegar mixture; let cool slightly.

3. Transfer to an airtight container and store in the refrigerator for up to 1 week.

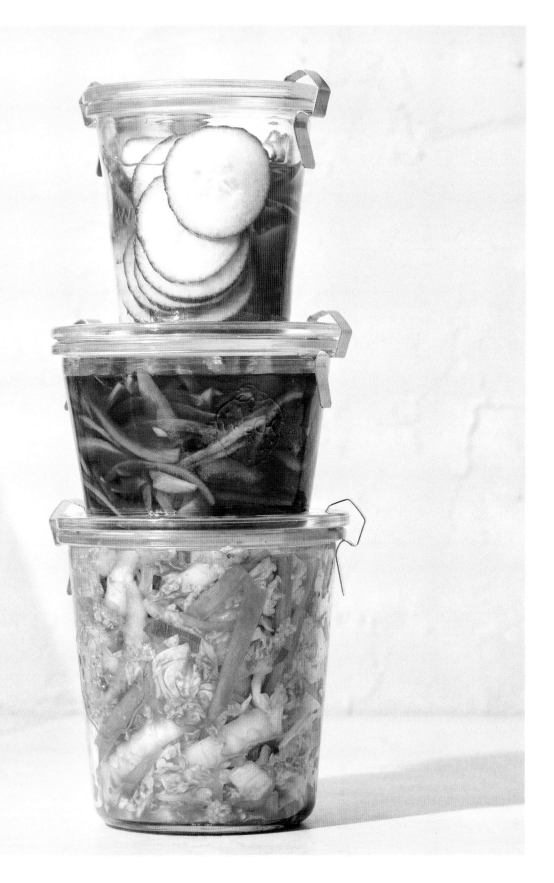

Quick Pickled Cucumbers

Makes: 2 cups

Prep Time: 30 minutes, including chilling time

2 cups thinly sliced English cucumber

1 teaspoon kosher salt

⅔ cup rice wine vinegar

This is a ready-to-eat pickle, meaning it can't be stored for long: It keeps in the fridge for a day or two at most. Feel free to add chiles, peppercorns, or any other spices to the pickling liquid to enhance the flavor.

Place the cucumber in a large bowl. Add the salt and vinegar and mix well until everything is fully coated. Transfer to an airtight container and refrigerate for at least 30 minutes before serving.

Quick "Kimchi"

Makes: 2 cups

Prep Time: 20 minutes

1 small napa cabbage, outer leaves removed, shredded

1 cup sliced scallions

1 large carrot, peeled and julienned

1 teaspoon kosher salt

2 tablespoons gochujang paste

1 tablespoon fish sauce

1 tablespoon rice wine vinegar

2 teaspoons maple syrup

1 (1-inch) piece fresh ginger, peeled and grated

1 garlic clove, grated

1 teaspoon gluten-free tamari

This "kimchi" has all the delicious flavors of traditional kimchi, yet takes only about 20 minutes to make. It's spicy, umami, and crunchy, making it the perfect condiment for eggs, rice, chicken, or fish.

1. In a large colander, combine the cabbage, scallions, and carrot. Sprinkle the salt all over and massage into the vegetables. Allow the mixture to sit for 10 minutes. Rinse the veggies well, then dry them very well with a tea towel. Transfer to a clean bowl and set aside.

2. In a small bowl, stir the gochujang paste with the fish sauce, vinegar, maple syrup, ginger, garlic, and tamari. Add the paste to the cabbage mixture and mix well until fully combined.

3. Store in an airtight container in the refrigerator for up to 1 week.

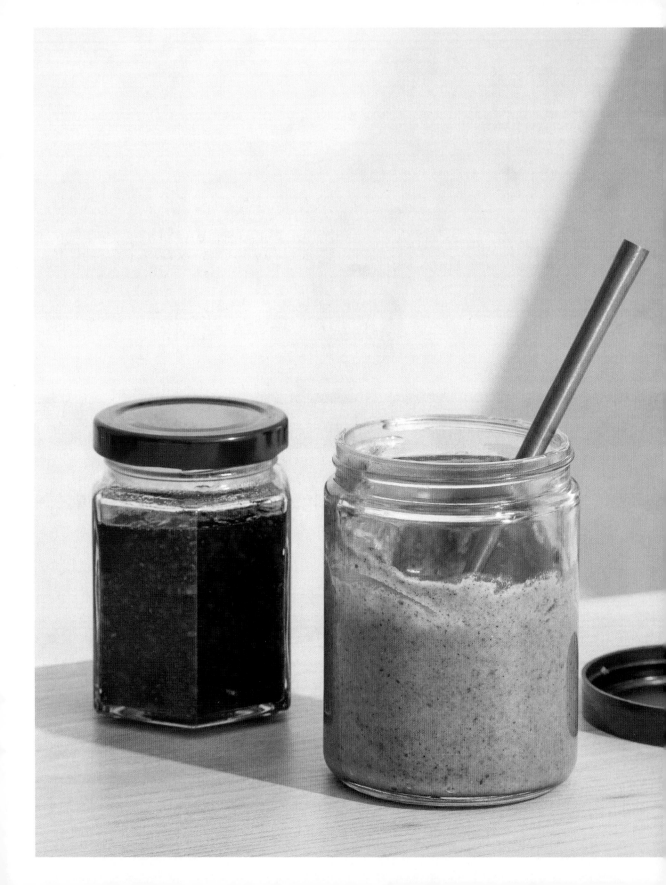

Hazelnut Almond Butter

Makes: 1 cup

Prep Time: 5 minutes

Cook Time: 10 minutes

1 cup skinned hazelnuts

1 cup whole raw almonds

1 Medjool date

Boiling water

1 teaspoon ground cinnamon

1 teaspoon vanilla bean paste
or vanilla extract

Pinch of salt

Homemade nut butters are quick and easy, and this hazelnut almond butter is about to become your new favorite. Both hazelnuts and almonds are packed with protein and fiber, making this a healthy spread to smear on crackers, enjoy with fresh fruit, or eat right off the spoon!

1. Preheat the oven to 350°F.

2. Place the hazelnuts and almonds on a baking sheet and bake, shaking the pan a few times to ensure even cooking, for 8 to 10 minutes, until golden.

3. Place the date in a heatproof bowl, cover with just boiled water, and soak for 5 minutes, then drain.

4. Transfer the warm nuts to a food processor and blend until smooth, about 8 minutes, scraping down the sides as needed. Add the date, cinnamon, vanilla, and salt and continue blending for 2 to 3 minutes, until smooth.

5. Transfer to an airtight container and store in the pantry for up to 1 month.

Pumpkin Seed Cardamom Butter

Makes: 1 cup

Prep Time: 5 minutes

Cook Time: 20 minutes

2 cups raw pumpkin seeds

2 Medjool dates

Boiling water

1 teaspoon ground cardamom

1 teaspoon ground cinnamon

1 teaspoon ground ginger

2 tablespoons melted coconut oil

Highly nutritious pumpkin seeds are rich in antioxidants, iron, and magnesium, all of which contribute to better heart health and blood sugar regulation. Lightly spiced with warming notes of cardamom and cinnamon, this flavorsome pumpkin seed butter can be used in smoothies or stirred into yogurt.

1. Preheat the oven to 350°F.

2. Place the pumpkin seeds on a baking sheet and bake for 8 to 10 minutes, until golden, shaking the pan a few times to ensure even cooking.

3. Place the dates in a heatproof bowl, cover with just boiled water, and soak for 5 minutes, then drain.

4. Transfer the warm seeds to a food processor and blend, scraping down the sides as needed, until smooth, about 8 minutes. Add the dates, cardamom, cinnamon, ginger, and coconut oil. Continue blending for 2 to 3 minutes, until smooth.

5. Transfer to an airtight container and store in the pantry for up to 1 month.

Raspberry-Vanilla Chia Jam

Makes: 1 cup

Prep Time: 5 minutes,
plus 3 hours chilling time
Cook Time: 5 minutes

2 cups frozen raspberries

2 tablespoons chia seeds

1 tablespoon lemon juice

1 teaspoon vanilla extract

1 to 2 tablespoons maple
syrup, as needed

Raspberries are low-calorie, nutrient-dense, and low on the glycemic index. They contain a significant amount of fiber and vitamin C, which is essential for iron absorption and a strong immune function. They also contain strong antioxidant compounds that can help prevent disease. Delicious in jams, they add naturally tart and sweet flavors that pair well with nut butters and smoothies.

1. Cook the berries in a small pot over medium heat, stirring, for about 5 minutes, until broken down. Remove from the heat and stir in the chia seeds, lemon juice, and vanilla. Add the maple syrup to taste, depending how sweet the fruit is. Let cool completely.

2. Chill in an airtight container in the refrigerator for at least 3 hours before serving, best overnight. Store in the fridge for up to 2 weeks.

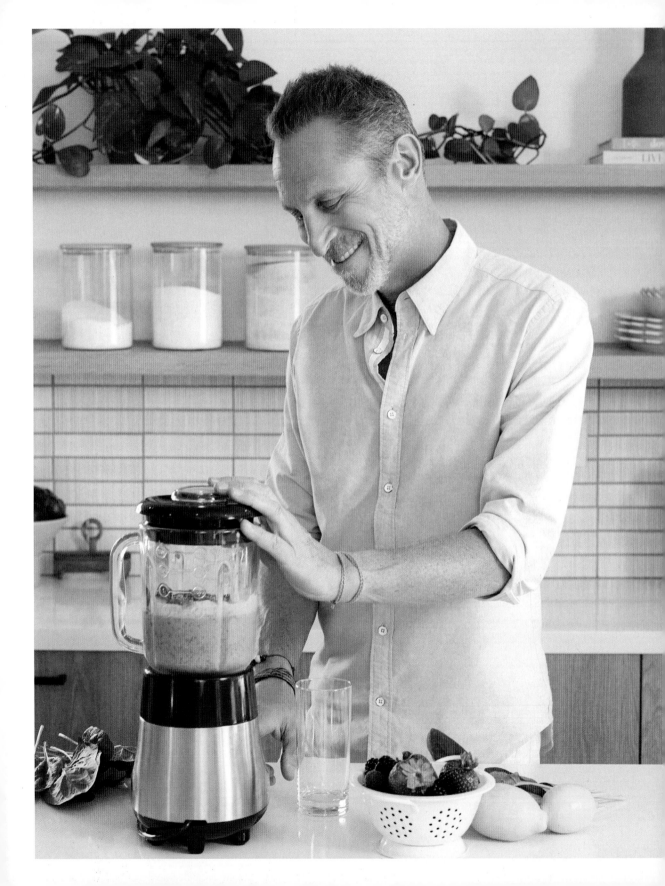

Blueberry-Lavender Chia Jam

Makes: 1 cup

Prep Time: 5 minutes,
plus 3 hours chilling time
Cook Time: 5 minutes

2 cups frozen blueberries

2 tablespoons chia seeds

1 tablespoon lemon juice

½ teaspoon dried lavender flowers

1 to 2 tablespoons maple syrup, as needed

Blueberries are such a wonderful berry, rich in the antioxidant anthocyanins, which give them their beautiful blue hue and can help reduce your risk of chronic disease. They also contain essential vitamins and minerals such as vitamin C and vitamin K1, which aids in blood clotting. Packed with flavonoids, blueberries have been linked with improved brain and heart health. Sweet and juicy, they are great to incorporate into your daily meals. Swirling this jam into a smoothie, or pairing it with a nut butter on some gluten-free toast makes that easy!

1. Cook the berries in a small pot over medium heat, stirring, for about 5 minutes, until broken down.

2. Remove from the heat and stir in the chia seeds, lemon juice, and lavender. Add the maple syrup to taste, depending how sweet the fruit is. Let cool completely.

3. Chill in an airtight container in the refrigerator for at least 3 hours before serving, best overnight. Store in the fridge for up to 2 weeks.

ACKNOWLEDGMENTS

Cooking is a revolutionary act. It empowers us with the skills and tools to take back our kitchens and our health. I learned to cook as a child with my mother in her kitchen using only the freshest ingredients (except for Tang, the drink of astronauts, but I forgive my mother because it was the 1970s after all). But many people need a guidebook. Think of this cookbook as a GPS system guiding you to a long healthy life, full of pleasure and yumminess.

Writing a cookbook is a team sport. I could not have done it without the help of the many people working behind the scenes. So many were instrumental in creating this book. Dara Sutin helped with recipe creation and was our amazing food stylist and culinary consultant. The beautiful photographs were taken by Kyla Zanardi, and the prop stylist and art director Rayna Marlee Schwartz made the dishes look as good as they taste. And of course, someone had to taste them all to make sure they were as delicious as possible. That human was Becca Pozner, who also helped with food styling. Some of the pictures in the book (including the ones of me) were taken by Masha Maltsava. Jessica Boone helped make the food in those pictures look so good. The nutritional analyses were done by Amy Hebert. Without this team of dedicated, creative, and exceptional artists, this book would not have come to be. Thank you, thank you, thank you.

And of course, the people from my own team, those who keep the ship running and make me look good, who put their heart and soul into the book, and who helped with the organization, planning, and coordination to help get this book out into the world are literally the best! None of this would have been possible without them. Thank you Darci Gross and Jennifer Sanders. Beyond grateful for you.

To my assistant Meredith, thank you for literally everything. Without you I would be lost. I'd also like to thank the rest of the Hyman Digital team for helping me share the power of real food with others. You are the best team in the world. In addition to Darci and Jennifer, I want to deeply thank Farrell Feighan, Lauren Feighan, Ailsa Cowell, Alex Gallegos, Patrick Edwards, Melanie Haraldson, Kay Lemus, Ayelet Menashe, Susan Verity, Linda Cardillo, Taylor Groff, Amber Cox, Mary Workman, Carol Syversen, Tammy Boyd, Dianna Towns, Mara Floyd, and Justin Johnson.

Of course, my team at The UltraWellness Center keeps the wheels on the bus when I am out working on all my books. A special thank you to Liz Boham, Todd Lepine, George Papanicolaou, Gerry Doherty, and the entire UWC staff.

I want to thank my team at Little, Brown for making this all possible. My editor, Tracy Behar, there from my first book to hopefully my last, has helped me make a bigger impact on the world than I ever imagined. My agent, Richard Pine, saw me as a young thirtysomething with bold ideas, took a flyer on me, and has been on this whole ride for more than twenty years. Thank you both.

Of course, my family—Rachel, Misha, Sarah, and Ben—give me such joy and have endured the sometimes-challenging ride. And my friends (it would take another book to name them all)—you know who you are and how much I love you and am grateful for your support.

To all the wonderful humans I have met on my journeys to the Blue Zones, thank you. The old and the young—you were such an inspiration for this book!

And last but never least, my life partner and human Brianna Welsh, who sees all, knows all, and still loves me sometimes better than I love myself. Thank you for being my home.

RECIPE INDEX

NUTRITIONAL ANALYSIS INDEX

RECIPE	NUTRITIONAL ANALYSIS
Almond Dukkah	Per ½ Cup Serving: Calories: 271, Fat: 23 g, Saturated Fat: 2 g, Cholesterol: 0 mg, Fiber: 7 g, Protein: 10 g, Carbohydrates: 11 g, Sodium: 602 mg
Antioxidant Berry Smoothie	Per Serving: Calories: 259, Fat: 3 g, Saturated Fat: 0 g, Cholesterol: 0 mg, Fiber: 12 g, Protein: 10 g, Carbohydrates: 55 g, Sodium: 83 mg
Arugula and Pumpkin Seed Pesto	Per ¼ Cup Serving: Calories: 208, Fat: 20 g, Saturated Fat: 3 g, Cholesterol: 0 mg, Fiber: 3 g, Protein: 3 g, Carbohydrates: 6 g, Sodium: 266 mg
Asparagus Vinaigrette	Per Serving: Calories: 239, Fat: 21 g, Saturated Fat: 3 g, Cholesterol: 105 mg, Fiber: 3 g, Protein: 7 g, Carbohydrates: 8 g, Sodium: 339 mg
Baked Eggs with Chickpeas and Tomatoes	Per Serving: Calories: 487, Fat: 25 g, Saturated Fat: 5 g, Cholesterol: 278 mg, Fiber: 14 g, Protein: 25 g, Carbohydrates: 46 g, Sodium: 1917 mg
Balsamic Marinated Steak with Broccolini	Per Serving: Calories: 677, Fat: 57 g, Saturated Fat: 14 g, Cholesterol: 70 mg, Fiber: 8 g, Protein: 26 g, Carbohydrates: 15 g, Sodium: 407 mg
Basil Walnut Pesto	Per ¼ Cup Serving: Calories: 347, Fat: 35 g, Saturated Fat: 6 g, Cholesterol: 13 mg, Fiber: 8 g, Protein: 2 g, Carbohydrates: 4 g, Sodium: 296 mg
Beef Kofte with Hummus	Per Serving: Calories: 404, Fat: 22 g, Saturated Fat: 6 g, Cholesterol: 67 mg, Fiber: 8 g, Protein: 27 g, Carbohydrates: 25 g, Sodium: 1053 mg
Beef Short Rib Ragu	Per Serving: Calories: 494, Fat: 20 g, Saturated Fat: 6 g, Cholesterol: 165 mg, Fiber: 7 g, Protein: 62 g, Carbohydrates: 21 g, Sodium: 1017 mg
Berbere Chicken with Tahini	Per Serving: Calories 1063, Fat: 45 g, Saturated Fat: 9 g, Cholesterol: 366 mg, Fiber: 5 g, Protein: 146 g, Carbohydrates: 13 g, Sodium: 1003 mg
Bison Meatballs with Braised White Beans	Per Serving: Calories: 568, Fat: 26 g, Saturated Fat: 5 g, Cholesterol: 137 mg, Fiber: 10 g, Protein: 47 g, Carbohydrates: 37 g, Sodium: 1257 mg
Bitter Greens with Steak and Romesco Sauce	Per Serving: Calories: 478, Fat: 35 g, Saturated Fat: 6 g, Cholesterol: 87 mg, Fiber: 2 g, Protein: 37 g, Carbohydrates: 7 g, Sodium: 890 mg

Black Bean Soup with Tomato Salsa	Per Serving: Calories: 584, Fat: 13 g, Saturated Fat: 2 g, Cholesterol: 0 mg, Fiber: 38 g, Protein: 28 g, Carbohydrates: 94 g, Sodium: 2030 mg
Blackberry and Mint Refresher	Per Serving: Calories: 59, Fat: 0 g, Saturated Fat: 0 g, Cholesterol: 0 mg, Fiber: 5 g, Protein: 2 g, Carbohydrates: 16 g, Sodium: 3 mg
Blueberry-Lavender Chia Jam	Per Serving: Calories: 328, Fat: 7 g, Saturated Fat: 1 g, Cholesterol: 0 mg, Fiber: 14 g, Protein: 6 g, Carbohydrates: 9 g, Sodium: 68 mg
Braised Pomegranate Lamb Shanks	Per Serving: Calories: 976, Fat: 53 g, Saturated Fat: 17 g, Cholesterol: 299 mg, Fiber: 2 g, Protein: 90 g, Carbohydrates: 21 g, Sodium: 994 mg
Broccoli and Quinoa Slaw with Wild Salmon and Hemp Pesto	Per Serving: Calories: 681, Fat: 38 g, Saturated Fat: 5 g, Cholesterol: 38 mg, Fiber: 5 g, Protein: 32 g, Carbohydrates: 61 g, Sodium: 547 mg
Brussels Sprouts with Pecorino and Hazelnuts	Per Serving: Calories: 260, Fat: 20 g, Saturated Fat: 4 g, Cholesterol: 13 mg, Fiber: 5 g, Protein: 9 g, Carbohydrates: 14 g, Sodium: 733 mg
Buckwheat Bowl with Smoked Paprika Chicken	Per Serving: Calories: 707, Fat: 36 g, Saturated Fat: 6 g, Cholesterol: 104 mg, Fiber: 14 g, Protein: 51 g, Carbohydrates: 50 g, Sodium: 1165 mg
Butternut Squash Curry with Cucumber Relish	Per Serving: Calories: 624, Fat: 32 g, Saturated Fat: 17 g, Cholesterol: 0 mg, Fiber: 19 g, Protein: 15 g, Carbohydrates: 77 g, Sodium: 988 mg
Cabbage Slaw with Savory Seed Mix	Per Serving: Calories: 316, Fat: 21 g, Saturated Fat: 3 g, Cholesterol: 0 mg, Fiber: 7 g, Protein: 13 g, Carbohydrates: 24 g, Sodium: 548 mg
Caramelized Carrots with Lime Yogurt	Per Serving: Calories: 172, Fat: 8 g, Saturated Fat: 1 g, Cholesterol: 3 mg, Fiber: 5 g, Protein: 8 g, Carbohydrates: 20 g, Sodium: 1101 mg
Cashew Hollandaise	Per ½ Cup Serving: Calories: 203, Fat: 15 g, Saturated Fat: 3 g, Cholesterol: 0 mg, Fiber: 2 g, Protein: 8 g, Carbohydrates: 330 g, Sodium: 13 mg
Cauliflower Gratin	Per Serving: Calories: 242, Fat: 14 g, Saturated Fat: 6 g, Cholesterol: 26 mg, Fiber: 7 g, Protein: 10 g, Carbohydrates: 856 g, Sodium: 23 mg

Cauliflower Rice Burrito Bowl	Per Serving: Calories: 490, Fat: 30 g, Saturated Fat: 5 g, Cholesterol: 0 mg, Fiber: 17 g, Protein: 15 g, Carbohydrates: 49 g, Sodium: 1083 mg
Chermoula	Per ¼ Cup Serving: Calories: 92, Fat: 7 g, Saturated Fat: 1 g, Cholesterol: 2 mg, Fiber: 0 g, Protein: 5 g, Carbohydrates: 3 g, Sodium: 170 mg
Chewy Chocolate Coconut Cookies	Per Serving: Calories: 182, Fat: 12 g, Saturated Fat: 5 g, Cholesterol: 27 mg, Fiber: 4 g, Protein: 4 g, Carbohydrates: 16 g, Sodium: 48 mg, Sugar: 7 g
Chicken Tortilla Soup	Per Serving: Calories: 398, Fat: 10 g, Saturated Fat: 2 g, Cholesterol: 96 mg, Fiber: 6 g, Protein: 42 g, Carbohydrates: 35 g, Sodium: 1289 mg
Chicken with Kale and Preserved Lemon	Per Serving: Calories: 389, Fat: 17 g, Saturated Fat: 4 g, Cholesterol: 194 mg, Fiber: 2 g, Protein: 45 g, Carbohydrates: 18 g, Sodium: 1349 mg
Chickpea Chop Salad with Whipped Jalapeño Feta	Per Serving: Calories: 472, Fat: 38 g, Saturated Fat: 10 g, Cholesterol: 51 mg, Fiber: 12 g, Protein: 21 g, Carbohydrates: 40 g, Sodium: 1613 mg
Chickpea Curry with Beet Raita	Per Serving: Calories: 233, Fat: 5 g, Saturated Fat: 2 g, Cholesterol: 0 mg, Fiber: 11 g, Protein: 10 g, Carbohydrates: 40 g, Sodium: 1613 mg
Chickpea Socca with Broccolini and Chermoula	Per Serving: Calories 231, Fat: 16 g, Saturated Fat: 2 g, Cholesterol: 0 mg, Fiber: 4 g, Protein: 7 g, Carbohydrates: 548 g, Sodium: 16 mg
Chipotle Bison Chili	Per Serving: Calories: 493, Fat: 18 g, Saturated Fat: 6 g, Cholesterol: 83 mg, Fiber: 10 g, Protein: 42 g, Carbohydrates: 40 g, Sodium: 1151 mg
Coconut and Chocolate Blueberry Clusters	Per Serving: Calories: 212, Fat: 18 g, Saturated Fat: 11 g, Cholesterol: 0 mg, Fiber: 4 g, Protein: 2 g, Carbohydrates: 16 g, Sodium: 7 mg, Sugar: 8 g
Coconut Carrot Soup with Crispy Chickpeas	Per Serving: Calories: 594, Fat: 33 g, Saturated Fat: 17 g, Cholesterol: 0 mg, Fiber: 17 g, Protein: 14 g, Carbohydrates: 65 g, Sodium: 1724 mg
Coconut Cobb Salad	Per Serving: Calories 420, Fat: 33 g, Saturated Fat: 15 g, Cholesterol: 185 mg, Fiber: 7 g, Protein: 11 g, Carbohydrates: 23 g, Sodium: 872 mg

Coconut Matcha Popsicles	Per Serving: Calories: 125, Fat: 10 g, Saturated Fat: 9 g, Cholesterol: 0 mg, Fiber: 0 g, Protein: 1 g, Carbohydrates: 7 g, Sodium: 39 mg
Cold Soba Noodle Salad with Mushrooms, Bok Choy, and Tofu	Per Serving: Calories: 481, Fat: 30 g, Saturated Fat: 3 g, Cholesterol: 0 mg, Fiber: 10 g, Protein: 28 g, Carbohydrates: 37 g, Sodium: 962 mg
Creamy Almond Masala Chai Latte	Full Recipe: Calories 300, Fat: 17 g, Saturated Fat: 2 g, Cholesterol: 0 mg, Fiber: 14 g, Protein: 7 g, Carbohydrates: 37 g, Sodium: 235 mg
Creamy Zucchini Bean Soup	Per Serving: Calories: 248, Fat: 14 g, Saturated Fat: 2 g, Cholesterol: 0 mg, Fiber: 7 g, Protein: 9 g, Carbohydrates: 27 g, Sodium: 982 mg
Curried Butternut Squash Soup	Per Serving: Calories: 255, Fat: 10 g, Saturated Fat: 4 g, Cholesterol: 0 mg, Fiber: 6 g, Protein: 7 g, Carbohydrates: 40 g, Sodium: 610 mg
Dark Chocolate Seaweed Rounds	Per 3 Cookies: Calories: 146, Fat: 11 g, Saturated Fat: 6 g, Cholesterol: 0 mg, Fiber: 3 g, Protein: 2 g, Carbohydrates: 10 g, Sodium: 156 mg, Sugar: 5 g
Edamame and Bean Salad with Crispy Tofu	Per Serving: Calories: 378, Fat: 24 g, Saturated Fat: 3 g, Cholesterol: 0 mg, Fiber: 7 g, Protein: 21 g, Carbohydrates: 561 g, Sodium: 25 mg
Egg Snack Pots: Avocado, Chili, and Lime	Per Serving: Calories: 172, Fat: 13 g, Saturated Fat: 3 g, Cholesterol: 187 mg, Fiber: 4 g, Protein: 8 g, Carbohydrates: 30 g, Sodium: 184 mg
Egg Snack Pots: Hummus and Almond Dukkah	Per Serving: Calories: 168, Fat: 12 g, Saturated Fat: 3 g, Cholesterol: 185 mg, Fiber: 2 g, Protein: 9 g, Carbohydrates: 6 g, Sodium: 252 mg
Egg Snack Pots: Spicy Harissa and Yogurt	Per Serving: Calories: 98, Fat: 6 g, Saturated Fat: 2 g, Cholesterol: 187 mg, Fiber: 0 g, Protein: 9 g, Carbohydrates: 3 g, Sodium: 310 mg
Fennel Minestrone	Per Serving: Calories: 162, Fat: 4 g, Saturated Fat: 1 g, Cholesterol: 0 mg, Fiber: 8 g, Protein: 7 g, Carbohydrates: 28 g, Sodium: 1158 mg
Forbidden Rice and Salmon Poke Bowl	Per Serving: Calories: 487, Fat: 14 g, Saturated Fat: 3 g, Cholesterol: 26 mg, Fiber: 4 g, Protein: 29 g, Carbohydrates: 60 g, Sodium: 1242 mg

Ginger and Cashew Energy Balls	Per 3 Balls: Calories: 367, Fat: 25 g, Saturated Fat: 4 g, Cholesterol: 0 mg, Fiber: 4 g, Protein: 11 g, Carbohydrates: 32 g, Sodium: 11 mg
Goji and Coconut Trail Mix	Per ½ Cup Serving: Calories: 351, Fat: 28 g, Saturated Fat: 8 g, Cholesterol: 0 mg, Fiber: 19 g, Protein: 7 g, Carbohydrates: 19 g, Sodium: 115 mg, Sugar: 10 g
Harissa	Per Serving: Calories: 367, Fat: 34 g, Saturated Fat: 5 g, Cholesterol: 0 mg, Fiber: 7 g, Protein: 4 g, Carbohydrates: 18 g, Sodium: 1941 mg
Harissa Chickpea Stew	Per Serving: Calories: 286, Fat: 5 g, Saturated Fat: 1 g, Cholesterol: 0 mg, Fiber: 13 g, Protein: 10 g, Carbohydrates: 52 g, Sodium: 1270 mg
Hazelnut Almond Butter	Full Recipe: Calories: 1553, Fat: 135 g, Saturated Fat: 10 g, Cholesterol: 0 mg, Fiber: 30 g, Protein: 10 g, Carbohydrates: 67 g, Sodium: 2 mg, Sugar: 17 g
Hibiscus and Rose Refresher	Per Serving: Calories: 65, Fat: 0 g, Saturated Fat: 0 g, Cholesterol: 0 mg, Fiber: 0 g, Protein: 0 g, Carbohydrates: 17 g, Sodium: 3 mg, Sugar: 13 g
Himalayan Tartary Buckwheat and Berry Pancakes	Per Serving: Calories: 514, Fat: 25 g, Saturated Fat: 4 g, Cholesterol: 101 mg, Fiber: 8 g, Protein: 15 g, Carbohydrates: 65 g, Sodium: 237 mg
Homemade Nut Milk	Full Recipe: Calories, 524, Fat: 44 g, Saturated Fat: 16 g, Cholesterol: 0 mg, Fiber: 9 g, Protein: 14 g, Carbohydrates: 26 g, Sodium: 13 mg
Iced Matcha Lemonade	Full Recipe: Calories: 121, Fat: 0 g, Saturated Fat: 0 g, Cholesterol: 0 mg, Fiber: 0 g, Protein: 3 g, Carbohydrates: 28 g, Sodium: 5 mg, Sugar 19 g
Kimchi, Egg, and Avocado Bowl	Per Serving: Calories: 763, Fat: 43 g, Saturated Fat: 8 g, Cholesterol: 372 mg, Fiber: 22 g, Protein: 30 g, Carbohydrates: 74 g, Sodium: 371 mg
Kombu and Mushroom Broth	Per Serving: Calories: 195, Fat: 5 g, Saturated Fat: 1 g, Cholesterol: 0 mg, Fiber: 14 g, Protein: 17 g, Carbohydrates: 23 g, Sodium: 1056 mg
Lemony Dill, Chicken, and Quinoa Soup	Per Serving: Calories: 652, Fat: 32 g, Saturated Fat: 9 g, Cholesterol: 0 mg, Fiber: 4 g, Protein: 70 g, Carbohydrates: 16 g, Sodium: 1275 mg

Lentil and Spinach Salad with Spiced Chicken	Per Serving: Calories: 534, Fat: 24 g, Saturated Fat: 3 g, Cholesterol: 105 mg, Fiber: 10 g, Protein: 60 g, Carbohydrates: 30 g, Sodium: 740 mg
Matcha Vanilla Latte	Per Serving: Calories: 97, Fat: 3 g, Saturated Fat: 0 g, Cholesterol: 0 mg, Fiber: 1 g, Protein: 11 g, Carbohydrates: 6 g, Sodium: 170 mg
Mixed Berry and Almond Crisp	Per Serving: Calories: 378, Fat: 23 g, Saturated Fat: 11 g, Cholesterol: 43 mg, Fiber: 6 g, Protein: 6 g, Carbohydrates: 40 g, Sodium: 6 mg, Sugar: 14 g
Mushroom, Lentil, and Parsnip Rosti	Per Serving: Calories: 329, Fat: 13 g, Saturated Fat: 2 g, Cholesterol: 46 mg, Fiber: 9 g, Protein: 10 g, Carbohydrates: 45 g, Sodium: 1268 mg
Mushroom Stroganoff	Per Serving: Calories: 244, Fat: 8 g, Saturated Fat: 2 g, Cholesterol: 0 mg, Fiber: 5 g, Protein: 15 g, Carbohydrates: 27 g, Sodium: 643 mg
Mushroom Tapenade	Per Serving: Calories: 234, Fat: 22 g, Saturated Fat: 3 g, Cholesterol: 0 mg, Fiber: 6 g, Protein: 7 g, Carbohydrates: 8 g, Sodium: 743 mg
Mussels with Lemongrass and Ginger Broth	Per Serving: Calories: 198, Fat: 8 g, Saturated Fat: 2 g, Cholesterol: 40 mg, Fiber: 1 g, Protein: 18 g, Carbohydrates: 13 g, Sodium: 647 mg
Nut Butter Protein Balls	Per 2 Balls Serving: Calories: 249, Fat: 19 g, Saturated Fat: 3 g, Cholesterol: 0 mg, Fiber: 5 g, Protein: 12 g, Carbohydrates: 11 g, Sodium: 3 mg
Olive Oil and Almond Cake	Per Serving: Calories 376, Fat: 34 g, Saturated Fat: 4 g, Cholesterol: 93 mg, Fiber: 4 g, Protein: 11 g, Carbohydrates: 12 g, Sodium: 200 mg
Oven-Baked Miso Kale Chips	Per 2 Cups Serving: Calories: 126, Fat: 6 g, Saturated Fat: 1 g, Cholesterol: 0 mg, Fiber: 4 g, Protein: 6 g, Carbohydrates: 15 g, Sodium: 487 mg
Paleo Trail-Mix Muffins	Per Serving: Calories: 237, Fat: 18 g, Saturated Fat: 2 g, Cholesterol: 31 mg, Fiber: 4 g, Protein: 7 g, Carbohydrates: 16 g, Sodium: 187 mg
Pan-Roasted Zucchini with Lemony Herb Pesto	Per Serving: Calories: 198, Fat: 15 g, Saturated Fat: 2 g, Cholesterol: 0 mg, Fiber: 4 g, Protein: 5 g, Carbohydrates: 14 g, Sodium: 507 mg

Pickled Red Onions	Per 1 Cup Serving: Calories 50, Fat: 0 g, Saturated Fat: 0 g, Cholesterol: 0 mg, Fiber: 1 g, Protein: 1 g, Carbohydrates: 9 g, Sodium: 1777 mg
Pistachio Mint Pesto	Per ¼ Cup Serving: Calories: 343, Fat: 33 g, Saturated Fat: 5 g, Cholesterol: 0 mg, Fiber: 4 g, Protein: 5 g, Carbohydrates: 9 g, Sodium: 330 mg
Protein Powerhouse Smoothie	Per Serving: Calories: 421, Fat: 22 g, Saturated Fat: 3 g, Cholesterol: 2 mg, Fiber: 14 g, Protein: 26 g, Carbohydrates: 37 g, Sodium: 184 mg
Pumpkin Seed Cardamom Butter	Per ¼ Cup Serving: Calories: 440, Fat: 37 g, Saturated Fat: 11 g, Cholesterol: 0 mg, Fiber: 6 g, Protein: 18 g, Carbohydrates: 17 g, Sodium: 11 mg
Quick "Kimchi"	Per ½ Cup Serving: Calories: 89, Fat: 1 g, Saturated Fat: 0 g, Cholesterol: 0 mg, Fiber: 4 g, Protein: 4 g, Carbohydrates: 19 g, Sodium: 1207 mg
Quick Pickled Cucumbers	Per 1 Cup Serving: Calories 32, Fat: 0 g, Saturated Fat: 0 g, Cholesterol: 0 mg, Fiber: 1 g, Protein: 1 g, Carbohydrates: 4 g, Sodium: 1183 mg
Quick Spicy Tomato Soup	Per Serving: Calories 293, Fat: 15 g, Saturated Fat: 2 g, Cholesterol: 0 mg, Fiber: 10 g, Protein: 12 g, Carbohydrates: 32 g, Sodium: 1196 mg
Quinoa, Cashew, and Dark Chocolate Squares	Per 4 Squares Serving: Calories: 452, Fat: 29 g, Saturated Fat: 11 g, Cholesterol: 0 mg, Fiber: 5 g, Protein: 11 g, Carbohydrates: 41 g, Sodium: 103 mg
Quinoa, Strawberry, and Sunchoke Salad	Per Serving: Calories 407, Fat: 28 g, Saturated Fat: 7 g, Cholesterol: 25 mg, Fiber: 5 g, Protein: 11 g, Carbohydrates: 32 g, Sodium: 1147 mg
Raspberry-Vanilla Chia Jam	Per Serving: Calories: 300, Fat: 8 g, Saturated Fat: 1 g, Cholesterol: 0 mg, Fiber: 23 g, Protein: 6 g, Carbohydrates: 55 g, Sodium: 9 mg, Sugar: 25 g
Raw Chocolate Tart	Per Serving: Calories: 490, Fat: 34 g, Saturated Fat: 11 g, Cholesterol: 0 mg, Fiber: 15 g, Protein: 10 g, Carbohydrates: 42 g, Sodium: 4 mg, Sugar: 21 g
Red Lentil Tarka Dahl	Per Serving: Calories 455, Fat: 5 g, Saturated Fat: 1 g, Cholesterol: 0 mg, Fiber: 36 g, Protein: 30 g, Carbohydrates: 108 g, Sodium: 493 mg

Reishi Cacao Latte	Per Serving: Calories: 105, Fat: 5 g, Saturated Fat: 0 g, Cholesterol: 0 mg, Fiber: 4 g, Protein: 4 g, Carbohydrates: 12 g, Sodium: 221 mg, Sugar: 4 g
Roasted Beets with Lentils and Hazelnuts	Per Serving: Calories: 490, Fat: 40 g, Saturated Fat: 7 g, Cholesterol: 25 mg, Fiber: 11 g, Protein: 14 g, Carbohydrates: 29 g, Sodium: 773 mg
Roasted Cabbage Wedges with Tempeh "Bacon"	Per Serving: Calories: 254, Fat: 14 g, Saturated Fat: 2 g, Cholesterol: 0 mg, Fiber: 8 g, Protein: 11 g, Carbohydrates: 24 g, Sodium: 271 mg
Roasted Cauliflower Soup	Per Serving: Calories: 345, Fat: 23 g, Saturated Fat: 3 g, Cholesterol: 0 mg, Fiber: 7 g, Protein: 10 g, Carbohydrates: 29 g, Sodium: 1046 mg
Roasted Pepper Medley with Pine Nut Salsa	Per Serving: Calories: 302, Fat: 21 g, Saturated Fat: 3 g, Cholesterol: 13 mg, Fiber: 7 g, Protein: 9 g, Carbohydrates: 25 g, Sodium: 335 mg
Roasted Purple Sweet Potatoes with Dukkah and Tahini	Per Serving: Calories: 354, Fat: 16 g, Saturated Fat: 2 g, Cholesterol: 0 mg, Fiber: 8 g, Protein: 7 g, Carbohydrates: 47 g, Sodium: 736 mg
Roasted Red Pepper and Zucchini Frittata	Per Serving: Calories: 315, Fat: 22 g, Saturated Fat: 7 g, Cholesterol: 386 mg, Fiber: 3 g, Protein: 20 g, Carbohydrates: 10 g, Sodium: 1243 mg
Roasted Rhubarb-Strawberry Coconut Crumble	Per Serving: Calories: 400, Fat: 28 g, Saturated Fat: 24 g, Cholesterol: 0 mg, Fiber: 9 g, Protein: 5 g, Carbohydrates: 33 g, Sodium: 50 mg, Sugar: 9 g
Salmon with Fennel and Citrus Salad	Per Serving: Calories: 655, Fat: 40 g, Saturated Fat: 6 g, Cholesterol: 109 mg, Fiber: 9 g, Protein: 47 g, Carbohydrates: 30 g, Sodium: 598 mg
Salsa Verde	Per ¼ Cup Serving: Calories: 300, Fat: 23 g, Saturated Fat: 3 g, Cholesterol: 0 mg, Fiber: 2 g, Protein: 19 g, Carbohydrates: 5 g, Sodium: 4103 mg
Savory Breakfast Salad	Per Serving: Calories: 422, Fat: 34 g, Saturated Fat: 8 g, Cholesterol: 38 mg, Fiber: 3 g, Protein: 15 g, Carbohydrates: 17 g, Sodium: 747 mg
Seared Scallops with Bursting Tomatoes	Per Serving: Calories: 223, Fat: 12 g, Saturated Fat: 1 g, Cholesterol: 19 mg, Fiber: 4 g, Protein: 13 g, Carbohydrates: 18 g, Sodium: 1514 mg

Smoky Roasted Pepper and Walnut Dip	Per Serving: Calories: 418, Fat: 36 g, Saturated Fat: 4 g, Cholesterol: 0 mg, Fiber: 5 g, Protein: 8 g, Carbohydrates: 22 g, Sodium: 1468 mg
Smoky Scrambled Tofu with Chopped Salad	Per Serving: Calories: 278, Fat: 19 g, Saturated Fat: 3 g, Cholesterol: 0 mg, Fiber: 4 g, Protein: 12 g, Carbohydrates: 12 g, Sodium: 450 mg
Smoky Turkish Beef Kebabs	Per Serving: Calories 502, Fat: 28 g, Saturated Fat: 8 g, Cholesterol: 166 mg, Fiber: 1 g, Protein: 56 g, Carbohydrates: 5 g, Sodium: 457 mg
Soft Herb and Mushroom Omelet	Per Serving: Calories: 439, Fat: 39 g, Saturated Fat: 19 g, Cholesterol: 616 mg, Fiber: 1 g, Protein: 21 g, Carbohydrates: 3 g, Sodium: 1177 mg
Spiced Kohlrabi with Pomegranate and Feta	Per Serving: Calories: 216, Fat: 12 g, Saturated Fat: 4 g, Cholesterol: 19 mg, Fiber: 10 g, Protein: 8 g, Carbohydrates: 23 g, Sodium: 430 mg
Spice-Roasted Leg of Lamb	Per Serving: Calories 992, Fat: 65 g, Saturated Fat: 33 g, Cholesterol: 372 mg, Fiber: 1 g, Protein: 85 g, Carbohydrates: 3 g, Sodium: 883 mg
Spicy Edamame Hummus	Per ½ Cup Serving: Calories 263, Fat: 11 g, Saturated Fat: 1 g, Cholesterol: 0 mg, Fiber: 10 g, Protein: 13 g, Carbohydrates: 31 g, Sodium: 1004 mg
Steamed Fish with Ginger and Bok Choy	Per Serving: Calories 245, Fat: 11 g, Saturated Fat: 2 g, Cholesterol: 56 mg, Fiber: 1 g, Protein: 30 g, Carbohydrates: 6 g, Sodium: 1115 mg
Stewed Black-Eyed Peas with Swiss Chard	Per Serving: Calories: 230, Fat: 5 g, Saturated Fat: 0 g, Cholesterol: 0 mg, Fiber: 9 g, Protein: 12 g, Carbohydrates: 37 g, Sodium: 295 mg
Strawberry and Basil Refresher	Per Serving: Calories: 79, Fat: 0 g, Saturated Fat: 0 g, Cholesterol: 0 mg, Fiber: 4 g, Protein: 2 g, Carbohydrates: 22 g, Sodium: 4 mg, Sugar: 10 g
Summer Tomato Salad with Smoked Mackerel	Per Serving: Calories: 335, Fat: 21 g, Saturated Fat: 3 g, Cholesterol: 25 mg, Fiber: 6 g, Protein: 17 g, Carbohydrates: 25 g, Sodium: 956 mg
Super-Matcha Smoothie	Per Serving: Calories: 294, Fat: 13 g, Saturated Fat: 2 g, Cholesterol: 0 mg, Fiber: 7 g, Protein: 13 g, Carbohydrates: 37 g, Sodium: 174 mg

Nutritional Analysis Index

Super-Seed Quinoa Crackers	Per 4-7 Crackers: Calories: 268, Fat: 17 g, Saturated Fat: 2 g, Cholesterol: 0 mg, Fiber: 7 g, Protein: 11 g, Carbohydrates: 22 g, Sodium: 244 mg
Sweet Potato and Egg Stacks	Per Serving: Calories: 259, Fat: 17 g, Saturated Fat: 3 g, Cholesterol: 185 mg, Fiber: 5 g, Protein: 17 g, Carbohydrates: 20 g, Sodium: 395 mg
Tempeh Sausage with Eggs and Roasted Tomatoes	Per Serving: Calories: 347, Fat: 25 g, Saturated Fat: 5 g, Cholesterol: 185 mg, Fiber: 5 g, Protein: 20 g, Carbohydrates: 15 g, Sodium: 580 mg
Tex-Mex Breakfast Bake	Per Serving: Calories: 250, Fat: 14 g, Saturated Fat: 3 g, Cholesterol: 285 mg, Fiber: 3 g, Protein: 15 g, Carbohydrates: 16 g, Sodium: 1052 mg
Thai-Style Shrimp with Mango Salad	Per Serving: Calories: 663, Fat: 41 g, Saturated Fat: 13 g, Cholesterol: 214 mg, Fiber: 10 g, Protein: 36 g, Carbohydrates: 47 g, Sodium: 463 mg
Thai Turkey Larb Lettuce Wraps	Per Serving: Calories: 330, Fat: 20 g, Saturated Fat: 5 g, Cholesterol: 120 mg, Fiber: 2 g, Protein: 30 g, Carbohydrates: 8 g, Sodium: 823 mg
Tomato and Sardine Crisps	Per Serving: Calories: 298, Fat: 22 g, Saturated Fat: 5 g, Cholesterol: 31 mg, Fiber: 5 g, Protein: 15 g, Carbohydrates: 452 g, Sodium: 9 mg
Tomato Fish Curry with Coconut Rice	Per Serving: Calories: 826, Fat: 38 g, Saturated Fat: 19 g, Cholesterol: 71 mg, Fiber: 8 g, Protein: 37 g, Carbohydrates: 80 g, Sodium: 594 mg
Trail-Mix Energy Cookies	Per 1 Cookie Serving: Calories: 231, Fat: 18 g, Saturated Fat: 3 g, Cholesterol: 22 mg, Fiber: 3 g, Protein: 6 g, Carbohydrates: 14 g, Sodium: 113 mg
Tulsi Tea Lemonade	Per Serving: Calories: 65, Fat: 0 g, Saturated Fat: 0 g, Cholesterol: 0 mg, Fiber: 0 g, Protein: 0 g, Carbohydrates: 17 g, Sodium: 3 mg, Sugar: 13 g
Ultimate Recovery Smoothie	Per Serving: Calories: 308, Fat: 20 g, Saturated Fat: 9 g, Cholesterol: 0 mg, Fiber: 5 g, Protein: 6 g, Carbohydrates: 31 g, Sodium: 28 mg
Vegan Broccoli and "Cheese" Soup	Per Serving: Calories: 327, Fat: 18 g, Saturated Fat: 3 g, Cholesterol: 0 mg, Fiber: 10 g, Protein: 19 g, Carbohydrates: 30 g, Sodium: 946 mg

Vietnamese Turkey Bun Cha	Per Serving: Calories: 335, Fat: 21 g, Saturated Fat: 5 g, Cholesterol: 80 mg, Fiber: 3 g, Protein: 23 g, Carbohydrates: 15 g, Sodium: 883 mg
Wild Rice Bowl with Smoked Trout and Coconut Cucumber Salad	Per Serving: Calories: 400, Fat: 27 g, Saturated Fat: 16 g, Cholesterol: 37 mg, Fiber: 7 g, Protein: 17 g, Carbohydrates: 26 g, Sodium: 375 mg
Zucchini Ribbons with Grilled Chicken and Preserved Lemon	Per Serving: Calories: 298, Fat: 15 g, Saturated Fat: 2 g, Cholesterol: 70 mg, Fiber: 5 g, Protein: 30 g, Carbohydrates: 17 g, Sodium: 481 mg

GENERAL INDEX

Note: Page references in *italics* indicate photographs.

lime
  Blackberry and Mint Refresher, 171
  Caramelized Carrots with Lime Yogurt, *150*, 151
  Strawberry and Basil Refresher, 175

M

Mackerel, Smoked, Summer Tomato Salad with, *60*, 61
mango
  Forbidden Rice and Salmon Poke Bowl, 68, *69*
  Super-Matcha Smoothie, 21
  Thai-Style Shrimp with Mango Salad, *124*, 124–25
matcha powder
  Coconut Matcha Popsicles, 194
  Iced Matcha Lemonade, 172, *173*
  Matcha Vanilla Latte, 170
  Super-Matcha Smoothie, 21
meat, xxi. *See also* beef; bison; lamb
Meatballs, Bison, with Braised White Beans, 107
Milk, Nut, Homemade, 166
Minestrone, Fennel, *78*, 79
mint
  Blackberry and Mint Refresher, 171
  Cilantro Hemp Pesto, 51
  Pistachio Mint Pesto, *200*, 201
  Salsa Verde, 205, *207*
  Thai Turkey Larb Lettuce Wraps, *66*, 67
  Vietnamese Turkey Bun Cha, *110*, 110–11
  Whipped Jalapeño Feta, *56*, 56–57

mise en place, xvi
Miso Kale Chips, Oven-Baked, 36
Muffins, Paleo Trail-Mix, 34, *35*
mushrooms
  Cold Soba Noodle Salad with Mushrooms, Bok Choy, and Tofu, *72*, 72–73
  Kombu and Mushroom Broth, 98
  Mushroom, Lentil, and Parsnip Rosti, *144*, 145
  Mushroom Stroganoff, *138*, 139
  Mushroom Tapenade, *40*, 41
  Soft Herb and Mushroom Omelet, 8
  Tempeh Sausage with Eggs and Roasted Tomatoes, 12
Mussels with Lemongrass and Ginger Broth, *132*, 133

N

Noodle, Cold Soba, Salad with Mushrooms, Bok Choy, and Tofu, *72*, 72–73
nori
  Dark Chocolate Seaweed Rounds, *180*, 181
  Forbidden Rice and Salmon Poke Bowl, 68, *69*
nut butters
  Creamy Almond Masala Chai Latte, 168, *169*
  Ginger and Cashew Energy Balls, *29*, 29
  Hazelnut Almond Butter, *214*, 215
  Nut Butter Protein Balls, 26, *27*
  Quinoa, Cashew, and Dark Chocolate Squares, *184*, 185
nutritional yeast
  Cashew Hollandaise, 204

  Vegan Broccoli and "Cheese" Soup, 86, *87*
nuts, xix. *See also specific nuts*

O

oils, xvii
Olive Oil and Almond Cake, 182
olives
  Chicken with Kale and Preserved Lemon, *104*, 105
  Mushroom Tapenade, *40*, 41
  Seared Scallops with Bursting Tomatoes, 128
Omelet, Soft Herb and Mushroom, 8
onions
  Pickled Red Onions, 210, *211*
  Smoky Turkish Beef Kebabs, 112, *113*
oranges
  Olive Oil and Almond Cake, 182
  Salmon with Fennel and Citrus Salad, *122*, 123

P

Pancakes, Himalayan Tartary Buckwheat and Berry, *2*, 3
pans, xxiii
pantry ingredients, xvii–xx
paprika
  Berbere Spice Mix, 108
  Harissa, *207*, 208
parsley
  Chermoula, 206, *207*
  Gremolata, 141
  Lemony Herb Pesto, *160*, 161
  Pomegranate Gremolata, 116, *117*
  Roasted Pepper Medley with Pine Nut Salsa, *148*, 149
  Salsa Verde, 205, *207*

ABOUT THE AUTHOR

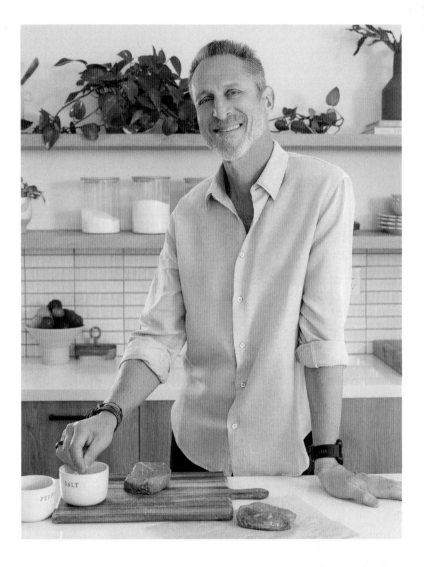

Mark Hyman, MD, is the founder and senior adviser for the Cleveland Clinic Center for Functional Medicine; founder and director of The UltraWellness Center; host of *The Doctor's Farmacy* podcast with more than 200 million downloads; cofounder and chief medical officer of Function Health; and author of fifteen *New York Times* bestsellers, including the #1 national bestseller *Young Forever.* Dr. Hyman received the Christian Book of the Year Award for his work on the Daniel Plan, a faith-based wellness initiative that he created with Rick Warren that helped the Saddleback Church collectively lose 250,000 pounds. He is founder and chairman of the nonprofit Food Fix Campaign, dedicated to transforming our food and agriculture system through policy.